W9-BGK-622

MRT

# MRT

*Walter Fischman C.M.D. and*
*Mark Grinims D.C.*

RICHARD MAREK PUBLISHERS

NEW YORK

First printing

Library of Congress Cataloging in Publication Data
Fischman, Walter Ian.
MRT.
Includes index
Bibliography
1. Food allergy—Prevention. 2. Muscle strength—Testing. 3. Orthomolecular medicine. I. Grinims, Mark, joint author. II. Title.
RC596.F57 616.9'75'075 78-15488
ISBN 0-399-90011-X

PRINTED IN THE UNITED STATES OF AMERICA

# Contents

# Acknowledgment

Many brilliant researchers have contributed to the various experimental sciences that form the base validity of MRT. We hope that this book will succeed in bringing the theories and concepts of these scientists to the general public so that a greater number of people may note, and benefit from, the significance and extent of their work.

Our deep gratitude is acknowledged to George Goodheart, D.C., who has devoted most of his professional life to discovering, rediscovering, testing, qualifying, and teaching the ever-expanding science of Applied Kinesiology.

We are also indebted to many others who are working, publishing, and teaching in the various aspects of this and related disciplines. Admittedly, the following list is only a partial one, but we hope it highlights a few of these dedicated physicians.

Terrence Bennett, D.C.
Richard Broeringmeyer, D.C.
Emanuel E. Cheraskin, M.D., D.M.D.
Major B. DeJarnette, D.C.
Walter K. Ehmann, D.C.
G.M. Ellison, D.C.
Carlton Fredericks, Ph.D.
K.R. McKillican, D.C.
Logan McKinsey, D.C.
Linus Pauling, Ph.D.
Robert J. Peshek, D.D.S.

Robert Ridler, D.C.
Herman Stoffels, D.C.
Fred Stoner, D.C.
John F. Thie, D.C.
David Walthers, D.C.

—Walter Fischman, C.M.D.
—Mark Grinims, D.C.

*New York, May 1978*

*To Emanuel Revici, M.D.,*
*with intense respect*
*and deep affection.*

—WF

*Respectfully dedicated to the memory of*
*my late brother*
*Henry Grinims, M.D.*

—MG

# Editor's Note

MRT works by means of a procedure known as muscle testing. As devised by Dr. Fischman and Dr. Grinims and presented in this book, it comprises a simple diagnostic method that the average person can readily use. But MRT is really a scaled down adaptation of another muscle testing technique. The parent science, called Applied Kinesiology, is vastly more complex in scope, application and interpretation. Intended for professional use, it is becoming recognized as a highly versatile, extremely useful healing modality.

# Foreword

Applied Kinesiology is the single technique that persuaded me to establish the concept of Transitional Medicine. Can you imagine a technique that allows you the opportunity of speaking directly to the body? Such a technique would enable you to ask almost any question, provided that the question is skillfully phrased in the body's language. Should a particular acupuncture point be treated? Is a certain herb right for a patient's condition? Is this abdominal pain from an ulcer or an inflamed gallbladder? Applied Kinesiology provides the ability to ask and answer these kinds of questions. Because of this ability, Applied Kinesiology is the major tool to build the transitional bridge between traditional medicine, dentistry and chiropractic and the plethora of new-age techniques that seem suddenly to have been thrust upon us.

As a technique, muscle testing is both general and specific in its application. How is this possible? It is general enough to be applied to all disciplines to ask questions about the appropriateness and effectiveness of any healing methodology from surgery to psychiatry. It is specific enough to ask the most detailed question about the finest points of any system in which it is applied. But, above all, muscle testing allows the practitioner to span disciplines, to see outside the confines of his or her own specialty, and begin to see the underlying principles that give life to all of the healing arts.

The principles of muscle testing are simple to learn and simple to apply, yet the concept is a more complex one than a superficial overview suggests. For one, muscle testing is a subjective experience between two people. This interaction implies cooperation, understanding and acceptance between the subjects involved. Modern medicine is uncomfortable in this setting. Where is the computer-precise objectivity, the demand for totally consistent results that could be performed equally by man or machine? Muscle testing reintroduces the human factor into medicine. It is this human factor, in my opinion, that will give dignity and ultimately effectiveness to the healing arts.

Secondly, muscle testing takes one into the realm of energy imbalance as the cause for disordered function. Western medicine is oriented to pathology—to looking at changes in body tissues after the changes have taken place, rather than trying to detect the process causing them. To me, this is like looking at the scoreboard after the game is over—it tells you who won but not how the game was played. You cannot change your strategy after the results are in. Muscle testing opens a whole new realm of body functioning on the dynamic level of energy relationship and here is where change can be effected.

Thirdly, the techniques of muscle testing will change the person who practices them. I have never seen this fail to happen. Whether doctor or lay person, one will find himself or herself no longer a mere observer but an active participant in the healing process. The person who is being tested and the person who is testing become engaged in a process of unraveling and balancing that demands a level of interaction that is both intimate and aloof at the same time. One might say that the energies of the two participants begin to work together like musical instruments in a duet. This interaction is the foundation for creativity and intuition.

Traditional medical practices are under a gentle pressure. The lay public is becoming more aware of the human needs that are left unassuaged by the complexity of modern technology. Doctors are now being asked to treat the patient's whole being. This change is not being induced by the insistence of a few idealistic individuals but is part of the changing age in which we live. Because this change is emanating mostly from the public and not from the professionals, I think we should welcome this book by Fischman and Grinims. Their book is an effort to introduce the first principles of muscle testing to the public. Such an effort will allow readers to help themselves in a very practical way, while simultaneously making them aware of their own uniqueness and complexity which must be respected when there is need to seek the expert guidance of their doctor.

JAS WANT SINGH KHALSA, M.D.

*Los Angeles*

# An Important Notice

MRT is intended to make you more aware of your own body and its intricate functions. If you use this book as it is intended to be used, the MRT process may bring you into a more effective relationship with the orthodox medical world.

The Muscle Response Testing technique that you can learn through this book will give you a fresh and potent viewpoint on your own physical and emotional well-being. Because it puts at your disposal a simple, easy-to-use way of maintaining an accurate check on yourself, you will know immediately when you are functioning below par. That's the time to call for help, not later when the medical problem has developed to the point that worse signs of ill health are evident.

You'll find that almost all doctors are delighted when they can stop potential health problems before they've had a chance to gain a foothold. Because you will, through MRT, have access to this "Early Warning System," you'll be in a position to cooperate more effectively with your doctor.

But even on your own, MRT can help you stay well and live your life with a degree of health that you may never have known before. Now, for the first time, you can literally fine-tune yourself, gradually trimming away the factors that are preventing you from enjoying optimum health. With MRT, it's easy to emphasize the beneficial elements, the subtleties that can be directed precisely at you, your needs, your wants, your life, your requirements.

But don't ever abuse this valuable tool. Self-diagnosis, even on a limited scale, can be a double-edged sword. If at any point you're not feeling well but can't track down a clue to the cause, do not hesitate to seek professional medical care. If you want the program to be truly effective, use all aspects of it . . . including the services of your family doctor.

MRT

CHAPTER

ONE

# What Is MRT?

As you know from the cover of this book, MRT stands for Muscle Response Test. Fine. But what's it for? Who needs it? Just what do those words mean?

MRT is an *indicator,* a simple, workable gauge that will give you a reading on the inner functioning of your own body. In effect, MRT is a window on your own well-being.

The procedure itself is simple. In a carefully controlled test situation, a muscle of your body is used to give a positive or negative answer to one of a number of questions about your physiological condition and requirements. In this manner, MRT can indicate which vitamins and minerals you need for your well-being and how much of each your body requires. MRT can also indicate whether or not you are allergic to specific foods and other substances. MRT uses the comparative strength of the test muscle to answer your questions. If the test muscle is strong, it means that you do *not* need additional quantities of the particular vitamin or mineral you have asked about; if the muscle is weak, it means you *do.* In the testing for allergies, a strong muscle means that you are *not* allergic to the substance being tested, a weak muscle that you *do* have an allergic reaction to that substance.

As contrasted with the standard diagnostic procedures, the complicated and costly laboratory tests and the vague and often unreliable evaluation of signs and symptoms, MRT is an accurate and revealing procedure that you personally can put into practice every day of your life. It may very well be the most significant tool you have within your reach to obtain and maintain optimum health.

Let's back up for a moment. We are not, by any means, suggesting that you abandon your family doctor or the procedures and medications of conventional medicine. Far, far from it. MRT is a process that will enable you to maintain closer contact with your own body, to achieve an awareness of its workings, as well as of its good and ill health. Properly utilized, it will help you become an informed patient. That means you will be able to work *with* your family doctor toward the mutual goal of your good health.

For the most part, MRT is designed to help you maintain optimum health. Once you get a working grasp of the technique, you'll be able to deal with a number of minor health problems *before* they assume major proportions. In this respect, you will be able to reach a level of well-being that you may never have known before. Should a more major health problem arise, however, you will be able to relate to your physician in a more meaningful way than you have previously been able. Why? Because you will be in tune with your own body; you will be able to give your doctor a more accurate report on your physical state than was ever possible in the past.

MRT uses no chemicals. No laboratory or special equipment is needed. It is not a medical procedure in the strictest sense of the word, although doctors throughout the world are themselves beginning to utilize the same methods you will learn in this book. Because of the level of their specialized knowledge, physicians can extend the tests further and draw more involved inferences from them than you can. Within the bounds of your own ability and competence, however, you can gain an entirely new and expanded insight into your own well-being.

Learning how to do it is surprisingly easy and incredibly swift. You don't have to put in years of diligent study in order to practice MRT. All you need are the instructions in this book, a brief practice session, and a friend to perform the actual testing. (Later you can turn the tables and do the same tests on your friend.)

Just what can you learn about your own health (or the lack of it) through the medium of MRT? For one thing, you can easily and accurately determine your body's vitamin and mineral requirements.

If you are like almost every other health-conscious person in the country, you are probably taking some sort of nutritional supplements. Again if you follow the norm, your whole "program" was undertaken on a helter-skelter basis and just sort of evolved in the course of time. It is quite likely that during this time you never once actually stopped to sort out what vitamins you really need. Instead you have fallen into taking various pills and potions in the hope that they would do you some good.

Most people are converted into a realm of health-consciousness through a similarly haphazard process. Let's say that you had a cold one day. A friend at work said, "You ought to try Vitamin C for that sniffle. You'll get over the cold faster." And maybe somebody else piped up with, "You should be taking Vitamin C regularly anyway. It will help keep you from getting colds, and it is the greatest for combating stress."

Stress? Colds? Talk about killing two birds with one stone! And anyway, what have you got to lose? Vitamin C is supposed to be harmless. If you take too much, you simply excrete it in your urine. And so on your way home that evening you stop at the drugstore.

At this point the routine gets a little complicated. There on the shelf you encounter ten, maybe twenty-five different types of Vitamin C. First, there's organic as opposed to man-made. There are the varieties with rose hips, not to be confused with the ones with Acerola, added. There are discount varieties and brand-name bottles. Is there a difference in quality? Maybe you would be better off with a combination tablet that contains other vitamins and maybe a dollop or two of minerals. Very confusing. So you ask the clerk behind the counter. Chances are he says something like, "Well, most of my customers use this," and he pulls a bottle off the shelf. Problem solved. You have made a choice.

But what kind of a choice? You are now taking the same Vitamin C tablet that most of the customers of that particular store are taking. But what does that mean? Stop to think about it for a moment. It may be a fine idea if your aim is to align yourself with the local average. But is that a reasonable goal in terms of your own well-being?

Hardly. You want what's best for your own body and the way you live with it. But in the absence of any reliable way of knowing what's best, you have been reduced to making a selection based on the opinion of a well-meaning friend compounded by the opinion of somebody behind the counter who probably never saw you before in his life.

So here you are, taking Vitamin C tablets on some sort of a schedule (probably the one printed on the side of the bottle). Your cold gets better (they always do eventually) but you continue the regimen to guard against the next cold.

Meanwhile you've noticed that some mornings when you get up, you feel a little achey and stiff in the joints. It just happens that a magazine you are reading contains an article that mentions that lack of calcium can sometimes be a causative element in a condition that sounds quite a bit like the aches that are giving you a touch of misery. Maybe you should take it as a sign. Come to think of it, the Vitamin C hasn't done you any harm so far; maybe it's even done some good. You can't tell for sure, but you think that you are perhaps not getting as many colds as before. Also, the day's turmoils don't seem to be getting through to you with as much impact as they used to. So the Vitamin C may be doing something . . . maybe. On that basis, maybe calcium could help your stiffness.

So it's back to the pharmacy where you go through the same routine and wind up with the same calcium tablets that most of the other customers are buying. Now you have a new schedule; you're taking two kinds of pills.

But things start getting a bit more complex. Perhaps the same nutritionally minded friend spots you taking your tablets one day at lunch and inquires what they are. "Calcium?" snorts your friend. "Your body can't use just plain calcium. It's totally useless unless you're also taking a balance of calcium, zinc, phosphorus, magnesium, and Vitamin D. Otherwise you're not getting anything out of the calcium."

Once more you head for the drugstore. At this point, you're a bit of an expert in your own right. You request the new pills by brand name. But once you've got them home, how do you know what dosage you should take? How much of one in proportion to how much of another will give you that all-important balance? Some of your pills are calibrated in mg (milligrams), some in IUs (International Units), and some in mcg (micrograms). How many micrograms make a milligram? Or is it the other way around—are milligrams divided into micrograms? And where do International Units fit into the picture?

It would seem only sensible to buy a book at this point. There is a whole shelfful at the health-food store, telling you how vitamins can open the door to vitality, health, longevity, and sexual strength. You choose one, and by the time you plow through the information contained in that single volume, you figure you should be taking enough tablets to stock several drugstores.

So you make a chart. One column for your total daily requirements, another for how those numbers can be divided up into the pills you should take at breakfast, lunch, and dinner. It's all quite precise, and your tally even takes into account some of the niceties you have learned, such as which vitamins cancel out which others, information you need to know so you can space them out from morning to evening.

The sum total of all those pills—the sheer physical bulk of it all—has now reached epic proportions. At lunch when you unwrap your baggie of assorted sizes, shapes, and colors of pills, a respectful hush frequently falls around you. Within your circle, it is generally known that you are on a megavitamin program. It is assumed that you are a walking powerhouse of health. With you, a germ wouldn't stand a chance.

Not that this notion of building the body so that it is impervious to the forces of ill health is a new one. In fact, one of the earliest comedy records included a variant of the old itinerant medicine peddler joke. According to his pitch, one of his customers drank a bottle of Indian Balm Liver Cure every day of his life. When he finally succumbed to the ravages of time at the splendid age of ninety-six, they couldn't bury him until they had cut out his liver and killed it with a club.

We're all seeking the same kind of armor at some level. We would like to be so healthy that no microbe or virus on the face of the earth could make headway with our bodies. We have, of course, far less than a fat chance, particularly if we persist in implementing programs of nutritional supplements on an irrational basis. On top of that, we are throwing money away.

Let's take a hard look at the pill-popping schedule we have been theorizing about. Does this really do you any good? Some . . . probably. For, in fact, very few people are in good enough physical condition that their bodies can satisfy all their nutritional needs from food intake alone. That's especially true of diets based on fast foods, junk foods, and the various other culinary disasters so popular today. So the chances are good that you need some sort of nutritional boost. And yes, it is reasonable to assume, in the case of some vitamins and minerals, that any intake above the precise amount that your body requires will be excreted automatically. But that's a long way from following a scientifically designed program tailored to your individual needs.

If you are seeking improved health through vitamin and mineral supplements, the only thing that will really work is a program custom designed for you: your needs, your body, and its ability to assimilate the contents of all those pills. There is a series of specific questions that must be answered before a personal nutritional program can be properly designed. The list includes:

1. Which vitamins do you need?
2. Which minerals do you need?
3. In what form should these be taken?
4. How much of each should you take?
5. Should you take your daily dosage of each all at once or in several smaller portions?
6. Should you take so-called organic (natural) or synthetic forms of the supplements?

7. Do any of the supplements work only or better if they are in combination with other supplements?
8. Do any of the supplements have a tendency to cancel out others when taken together?
9. Are there specific times of the day when the pills should be taken?

With MRT, you can answer each question on this list. What's more, you will wind up with a precise answer—yes or no, how much and when, no approximations.

But that's not all MRT can do for you. Because it works as a positive/negative gauge of the effect of external forces and substances on the inner workings of your body, MRT will enable you to check out many of the factors in your daily life that spell the difference between radiant good health and the "blahs," as well as out-and-out health crises.

Allergy, be it to a food or to a substance contacted by the skin, is an area in which MRT can be of enormous help. For virtually every human being alive, there are certain substances that set up an antagonistic reaction in the body. The allergen and the reaction vary markedly from person to person.

Most people think of allergic reactions, particularly to food, in terms of skin eruptions. The classic association is strawberries and hives. In fact, dermatological reactions are only one type of allergic manifestation, and not even the most common type. Much more frequent is the vague sense of being under par: no pep, no energy; in extreme cases, perhaps you doze off at your desk for a few moments at intervals during the afternoon. At home after dinner you may nod off in front of the television set. And quite frequently you just don't feel "up" for the parties, movies, sports and other social activities that contribute to the fun of being alive. This elusive feeling, this malaise, is often attributed to a whole range of things from low blood sugar to emotional problems, from vitamin deficiencies to the stresses of modern life. But did it ever occur to you that it might be a low-grade allergic reaction to something you ate?

To explain what we mean and how MRT can help pinpoint the problem area, let's take the case of a ham sandwich. Suppose every time you have a ham sandwich for lunch, you can barely make it through the afternoon. You never break out in hives or experience trouble breathing. Nothing as dramatic as that. You just feel lazy and not quite all there. Does that mean the solution is never to eat another ham sandwich?

No. The solution is to use MRT as a precise diagnostic technique, to isolate exactly which element in the ham sandwich is causing your distress.

It is possible that your unhappy reaction is caused by the bread. You can test this premise. You may find that you are allergic to rye bread but not white, to pumpernickel but not whole wheat. Or you may find that there isn't a single type of bread on the shelf that creates a problem for you. So maybe it's the butter. If not, there's a chance that the "butter" your local deli uses is really margarine, and that may be the causative factor. Check it out.

How about the mustard? Is it any mustard, or the specific brand or type of mustard on that sandwich? Maybe that thin sliver of lettuce on top could be the culprit, and just possibly it could be the ham itself. But does this apply to all types of ham, or is your allergic reaction to the chemicals used in curing the ham? The sugar coating around it? Do you have the same problem with baked ham as you have with boiled ham?

As you can see, a ham sandwich isn't all that simple. Through MRT, however, you can check out each individual component, each specific food that is a part of that sandwich. Come to think of it, you could even check the deli's take-out menu. There is a far-out possibility that you could be allergic to the plastic cover that protects it.

We could go on, but you get the idea. The point is that if you know you are allergic to something because you have a violent reaction every time you encounter a particular set of circumstances but you're not sure what individual element is responsible, MRT will permit you to identify the specific allergen. And if you aren't feeling as good as you think you ought to but you haven't any out-and-out symptoms that spell allergy, MRT will help you determine if allergy is the problem, and if so, what you're allergic to.

The same goes for what are commonly referred to as contact allergies, allergic reactions to substances that come in contact with your skin rather than being ingested.

Textiles represent a group of allergen suspects worth considering. Modern synthetics are commonly at fault, but it is certainly not unheard of to be allergic to natural fibers like cotton, linen, and even silk. With MRT you'll be able to check your response to any and all fabrics you come in contact with.

Allergic reaction can occur with various metals too. Some people cannot wear silver jewelry. With others, the problem occurs if they contact stainless steel. There is the classic case of an elevator operator who had a persistent skin irritation, which was finally tracked down to the brass control lever on the old-fashioned elevator he commanded. When this was covered with a leather sheath, his problem disappeared.

Cosmetics are a large and often troublesome category of potential allergens. If you suspect a problem in this area, your time would be well-spent subjecting the contents of each pot and bottle, stick and jar in your makeup arsenal to the MRT procedure.

As a matter of fact, anything that goes onto or into your body should be suspect. It is entirely possible that as a result of an MRT evaluation, you may have to change your brand of toothpaste, give away your dogs or cat, or stay away from the garden during pollen time. The choices are not always happy ones, to be sure, but with MRT you can zero in on the exact culprit and free yourself to enjoy the pleasures of an allergy-free existence.

You can even use MRT to check on such intangibles as the exercise program you are using to achieve a better physical condition. Should you be doing push-ups? Test yourself before and after. Are you doing too many of them? Test yourself after 10, 25, 50 or whatever number is in your regime. The same goes for jogging or running. Maybe one mile is what your body requires. Two miles might be fine, but three too stressful at this particular time. MRT gives the answer.

There's one factor to keep in mind no matter what you are

testing for. MRT will give you unequivocal answers but never an absolute answer good for all time. It is essential that you retest at regular intervals because your body does change. Left to its own devices, the tendency of your body is to get well. It tries to be strong, and there is a natural healing process that takes place unless something interferes with it. It is therefore entirely possible that you will slough off or outgrow a particular allergy, for example. Retesting is equally essential in the case of vitamin and mineral requirements. Once you have determined your need for a specific vitamin or mineral, be sure to retest every few months to determine whether that particular pill should remain in your schedule. It may be that as a result of the supplement, your body has developed the ability to produce the nutrient supplied by the pill. That's great; it's a process called getting well. When this happens, stop taking the pills.

MRT is a practical, predictable technique. It enables you to deal in absolute terms with the firm realities of your own body. With MRT, health is not a vague or elusive thing. It can be boiled down to a series of good or bad influences that you can positively identify and deal with in the most precise terms. We think that's a very exciting notion indeed.

CHAPTER

TWO

# Prove It to Yourself

In the previous chapter we made a series of strange promises; we offered some far-out hopes. Quite likely you are feeling a bit skeptical right now. That's good. No technique or treatment should be taken on faith alone. Its effectiveness should be questioned and then thoroughly proven before being accorded an ounce of validity. And that's what you should do with MRT. Right now.

Now is the time for you to prove to yourself that MRT really works. For MRT is real. It's a workable, usable, accurate technique. But you must be thoroughly convinced of this fact, as a result of your own direct experience, before we go any further.

MRT is a testing procedure that uses a muscle of your body as an indicator. The key word here is *indicator.* The muscle makes its indications by responding in different ways to different conditions. There are two responses: either the muscle is strong or it is weak; there is no middle ground.

The response is absolute, and absolutely clear. No interpretation is necessary and, except in the rarest of circumstances, there will be not a shred of doubt what the response is. We will discuss later how to handle those rare circumstances, of course, but in general you will have no trouble interpreting the responses you get.

Most of the MRT situations use a muscle called the deltoid, which originates at the shoulder and is responsible for moving the arm away from the body. Why use this muscle? There are several reasons: it's an easy muscle to identify, and it's equally easy to get at. It responds well and gives a clear indication of strength or no strength. In short, MRT uses the deltoid because it works.

It takes two people to put the MRT procedure into use, one to do the testing, the other to be tested. But unlike the traditional doctor/patient relationship or any of the numerous other superior/inferior setups, MRT works as a true equal partnership. Cooperation toward a mutual goal is part of it, but that can also be said of the best doctor/patient situations. The main difference is that with MRT you are both experts, both in touch with the body in question, and there is always the possibility that the tables will be turned, that tester will become testee.

In the course of much of the discussion that follows, our instructions will be addressed to the tester of the moment. The purpose, of course, is to clarify what one is to *do* in each situation. But an equally central participant in each of these cases is the one who is being tested, for indeed it is he (or she) whose health and well-being is, at the moment, the focus of all efforts.

Some of what follows may seem to you bizarre or just a bit silly. We assure you that there is a clear and rational basis for each action, and we will explain it all further on. For now, however, follow through the routine as detailed. Once you have seen how the procedure works, we can fill in with the reasons behind each aspect of the procedure.

There is a bit of preparatory work required. Both of you should be relaxed, so allow a few minutes' time to sit and unwind a bit. Although it is not essential that you be alone with your test-mate when you do MRT, you should ask anyone else who might be in the room to maintain a distance of at least two or three feet. And, of course, distraction should be eliminated. The atmosphere should be relaxed, though it need not be solemn.

Remove all metal from your bodies. The list includes watches, jewelry, pens, belt buckles, coins from your pockets. Don't worry about the eyelets in your shoes, but any larger metal items should be eliminated.

At the same time, it's a good idea to have the one of you who will be tested remove any article of clothing made from synthetic fibers—nylon, dacron, orlon, etc. This is not absolutely essential, but if it's not too much bother it will reduce the likelihood of anything interfering with the test procedure.

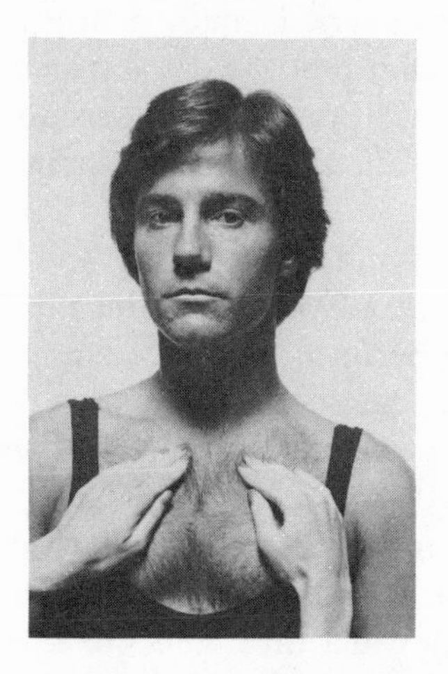

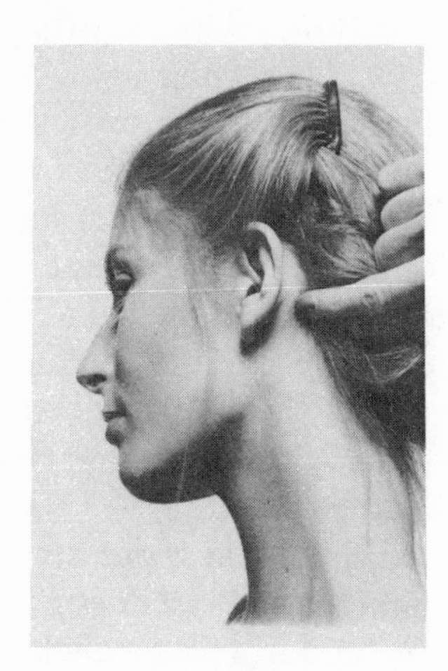

The next step is to neutralize the test subject. This is a two-step process that begins with rubbing two spots located just under the collarbone and one inch on either side out from the center of the chest. The collarbone, in case you're uncertain, is the long bone that runs across the top of your chest from shoulder to shoulder. The center is marked by a notch. Place your fingers one inch to the right and left of that notch and just below the bone itself. Massage with a circular motion, exerting fairly firm pressure. But do not push or poke your partner; the idea is to move the skin plus some underlying tissue. About fifteen or twenty seconds of massage will do the trick.

The second part of the neutralizing process involves massaging two other points, one located behind each ear. Place your fingers in back of the subject's ears so they rest on the bone that lies directly behind. Follow down until you reach the spot where the bone ends. This is the point we are looking for. Just make certain you are touching the point of the bone and not the hollow space below it.

In the same manner as you used on the points below the collarbone, massage these two points, pressing firmly and rotating the skin and a bit of underlying tissue for about fifteen seconds.

Finally, press the points behind the ear with your fingertips six or seven times without lifting your fingers. Employ a firm and rapid touch, exerting about three pounds pressure. (If you are not certain how much force this represents, press your fingers down on a bathroom scale first and try to recall, as you are neutralizing, the feel of that amount of force.)

The test begins with the subject standing or sitting and the tester standing facing him. It is generally easier if the subject stands as well, but if you decide to perform the procedure with the subject sitting, make certain that he does not cross his legs. For some reason, in some circumstances, this can interfere with the test results.

The subject leaves one arm hanging loosely by his side without touching his body (it does not matter which) and raises the other arm, palm down, to an angle slightly wider than 90 degrees; that is, the wrist should be a bit higher than the shoulder. The tester places the pads of his fingers on the top of the subject's wrist and, with his other hand, presses firmly on the subject's shoulder, thus stabilizing the subject's body.

In the course of the test, the tester will press downward on the subject's wrist while the subject resists that force. *Under no circumstances should this be a contest of wills.* The idea is to ascertain the baseline strength of the subject, not to determine which of the two of you is strongest. So forget the arm wrestling ethos.

The correct degree of pressure and resistance will be easier to maintain if you both follow these guidelines:

*Subject*—Keep your elbow straight.
Do not clench your fist.
Keep your fingers flat with the palm facing the floor.

*Tester*—It is inevitable that you will be the stronger of the two since your elbow is bent and your hand is closer to your body. This factor is built into the procedure.

Do not hang on the subject's arm; simply press down on his wrist against his resistance for a second or two. The force you apply should be smooth and progressive. The key problem here is how much force to use.

To help you gain a feel for this, you may find it useful as a training exercise to actually overpower a subject. Start off by establishing a base line of his strength. When he holds his arm up, tell him, "Resist me." Then press down, gradually increasing your pressure against his resistance.

If you are able to pull his arm down, it's a tip-off to the fact that you have exceeded his strength. From this point on, when testing this individual, use a little less strength. With practice, you won't have to overpower anyone but will be able to get a feeling for this strength during the two-second preliminary test.

If you are unable to overpower your friend, that's okay too. It just means that his strength is much more than yours. But you will still be able to use the procedure to gain a relative idea of his natural muscle force.

In either event, keep the feel of the force you applied in your mind so that you can relate to it again in the second half of the MRT procedure.

After you have tried out this exercise two or three times, you won't have to bother with it again. Instead you will be able to get a reading by pressing down for a couple of seconds without actually overpowering the subject.

Part two begins with a bottle of aspirin, the one-hundred-tablet size. The subject sticks his finger into the open bottle so that he actually touches the tablets inside. He can hold onto the bottle with his fingers as long as one digit remains inside touching the aspirin.

Repeat the muscle-test procedure, testing the arm that is not touching the aspirin. Follow exactly the same steps as before: test the same arm in the same manner. Tester and subject should stand in the same position; tester should, as before, place one of his hands firmly on the subject's shoulder.

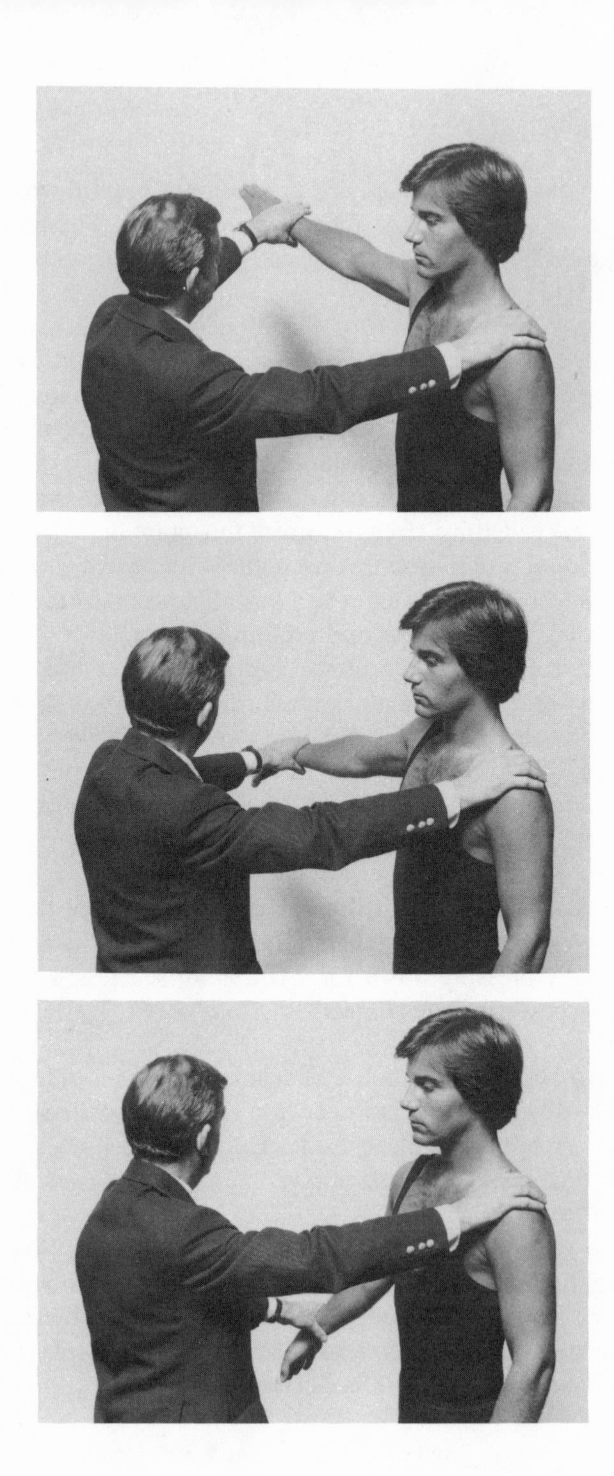

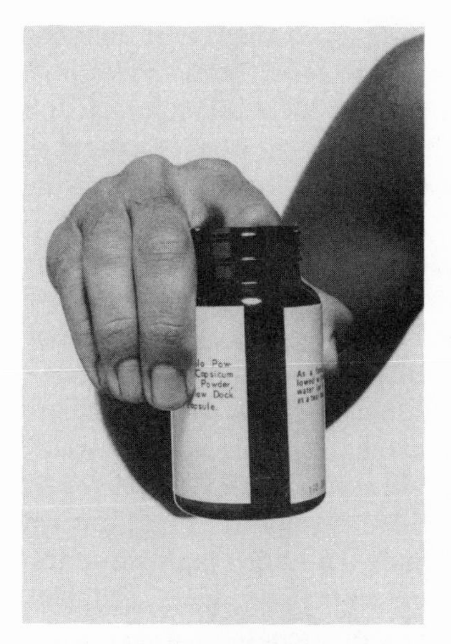

This time when pressing down on the subject's arm, the tester will notice a significant loss of strength. How much varies from person to person. The arm of some people will be so weakened that it will seem to drop almost of its own accord. There will be a small amount of resistance and then: down goes the arm. In others, the difference will be less dramatic, but still clear and unmistakable.

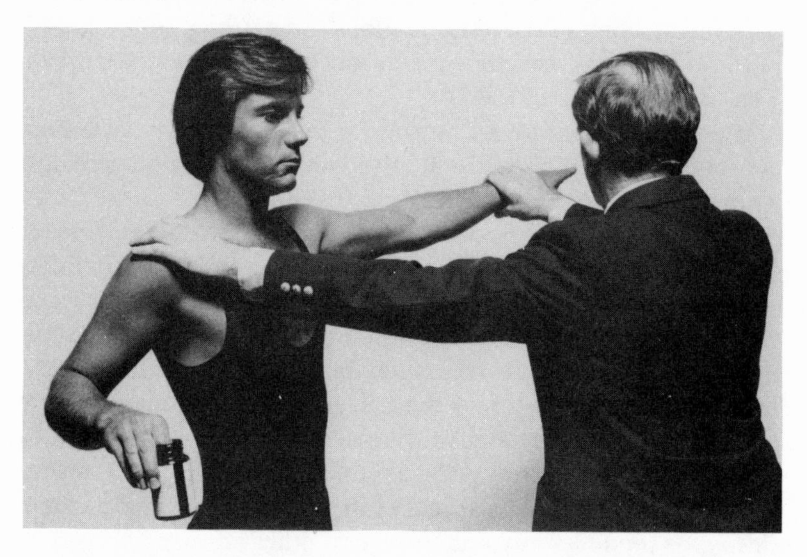

The subject should make an effort not to compensate. It's an eerie feeling to suddenly realize that the strength you had a few moments before is virtually gone. This makes some people very nervous, so instead of allowing it to happen they try to summon up the last reserves of their strength to resist. You should both understand that this is just a test and the effect is temporary. It is important that the test subject let his body do what is natural. If he attempts to distort the response, he is liable to shade the validity of the test.

Okay, so what happened? First, you got a reading on the subject's baseline strength. Then you introduced a poison. Poison? That's right. The aspirin. Aspirin in very large quantities is a poison. That's why it's sold with a child-proof cap, but the overdose danger does not apply only to children. If an adult were to take a whole bottle of aspirin at one time, the likelihood is that it would kill him too. One of the handiest things about MRT is that you do not actually have to ingest the substance you are testing. It is virtually as effective if you merely touch the stuff. That's why sticking a finger into the bottle of aspirin so that it touches the tablets is sufficient contact to give a reading of strength or weakness.

In the first half of the test, the subject was strong. In the second portion, when the aspirin was introduced, the subject was weak. That is the essence of MRT.

If you don't want to use aspirin for this preliminary test, there are other materials that will give you the same inequivocal strong/weak response. Just for fun, try chocolate.

But wait a minute, chocolate isn't a poison. Or is it? It depends on what you call a poison. If you mean something that will make you violently ill or cause you to fall down dead if you eat it, then chocolate is, of course, not a poison. But if you widen your definition to include any substance that can be harmful to the body, then chocolate fits well into this category. You see, many people are allergic to chocolate in varying degrees. Some know it—they may have learned from prior experience that chocolate makes them break out in hives, or makes them irritable, or makes them sleepy, or produces any one of several other adverse effects. For them, chocolate is a known poison. For most of the rest of us, even if we have had no such violent symptoms, chocolate does remain a hidden poison. If you ever get a craving for chocolate, you probably fall into this second group. For it's a sad fact of life that we seem to long for the foods that produce allergic reactions in us. Chocolate is one of the most common culprits.

Part one works just as we described in the aspirin test. Neutralize the subject and determine his baseline strength. Then have him chew a small piece of chocolate. While he still has it in his mouth, test a second time. In almost every instance, there will have been a noticeable loss of strength.

As an extra check on this, the subject should spit out the remains of the chocolate, rinse his mouth, and brush his teeth thoroughly. Wait two minutes to let the immediate effects subside. Then do part one again. The test muscle will have regained its baseline strength.

It's a pretty astonishing demonstration, isn't it? But more important, it is evidence of a precise and practical method for coming to terms with your own body. Through MRT, your body can speak to you in a language that you can learn to understand. Through MRT, you will gain an insight into the workings of your own physical mechanism. You'll see exactly how your body deals with the world in which you live, when it accepts and when it rejects, when it is helped and when it is harmed. It is all there for you to explore, and MRT is available to act as your guide.

CHAPTER
THREE

# Why Does It Work?

If you are seeking a neat, definitive answer to why MRT works, all we can say is, "We don't really know." Theories? Sure, we've got lots of theories and some of them seem pretty reasonable. But as for ironclad scientific proof . . . we're afraid not.

At least not at this juncture. A great deal of research is currently being conducted on the science of Applied Kinesiology, as well as the offshoot of it, which we're calling MRT. And it is hoped that at some time in the not too distant future, some dedicated researcher will come up with the answer. It's a bit like gravity.

A little over three hundred years ago, Sir Isaac Newton posited his theory of gravitation. As an explanation of a great number of natural laws, it worked very nicely and scientists have been depending on it ever since. But the fact is that today, on the brink of the twenty-first century, at the height of the age of space travel, we still do not know *how* gravity works nor *what* it really is. You may be comforted to know, however, that an inquiry into that is on the agenda of the scientific community and they hope to have an answer for us sometime within the next hundred years.

Felix Mann, M.B., has commented upon the process of acupuncture, which shares its philosophical framework with MRT. It works, it has worked for thousands of years, it has worked for millions of people, but nobody yet knows why. Says Dr. Mann, "A process which produces results but the principles of which we do not as yet understand is apt to be labelled as magic. Once it is understood, we call it science."[1]

Hopefully Applied Kinesiology plus such developments as MRT may help to restore soul to the cold practice of orthodox medicine.

This concept of caring is at the core of what has come to be known as "holistic" medicine. A patient is an individual, not a collection of systems and symptoms, and as such is much more than the sum of his parts.

We are witnessing the developing possibility of a new relationship between doctor and patient. More and more, they may be partners in treatment, jointly responsible for reversing an illness or promoting and maintaining good health.

MRT may be a signpost pointing in this new direction. For the first time, it is the patient's response that is the key factor in determining the therapeutic action taken. The signal originates within the person who is being treated and bears a direct relationship to his own body.

What about how it works, though? What progress has been made in understanding the theoretical basis of Applied Kinesiology and MRT? We must begin with the work of researchers in allied fields. For example, the likelihood is rather strong that MRT is effective because it operates on the energy pattern that exists on the surface of the body. The existence of this electrical field has been proven by Harold Burr, M.D. In the 1930s, Dr. Burr developed hypersensitive electronic instrumentation capable of reading electrical impulses in units as small as a millionth of a volt. Using this device, Burr discovered that there is considerable variation in the electrical charge present in different portions of a single body. He noted further that the voltage of the electrical charge varied greatly from day to day. Finally, he observed that different influences could change the electrical charge.[2]

Burr's work would seem to have some relevance in the area in which we are venturing. It seems likely that with MRT we are short-circuiting the flow of that energy. When you place your hand on a specific area of your body, or when the person testing you introduces a certain movement or action, the electrical charge is modified in some way. It's as though your body were acting as a sort of computer: it interprets the effects of or the need for a vitamin; it reacts to the toxic presence of a food to which you are allergic. Of course, it doesn't type out a report; instead this internal "computer's" readout is the weakening of a muscle.

The exciting thing about all this is that your body is the pivotal factor. The answers to all of these general health questions exist within your body.

Basically, there is nothing very strange about the whole idea of energy and the human body. After all, energy is all around us. It's there in the hot water flowing through the pipes in your house. In the kitchen it's there in an even hotter stove that's cooking your dinner. There's television and radio, static electricity, and sound. There's light and heat, X rays, ultraviolet rays, gamma rays. We are so accustomed to living with all of these energy forces that we take their presence for granted. We know that the energy is there and we accept the effects of it.

For example, when you tune in the eleven o'clock news, you are not aware of the energy that is passing through the walls of your house. It permeates the rugs, zips through the chairs, and finally passes right through your own body as if you didn't exist. And yet the only evidence you have of it is that it lights up the picture tube on your TV.

MRT is just such another manifestation of energy. And like the electrical energy that runs your television, you know it is there not because you can see or feel it in itself, but because you are aware of its *effect.*

The Chinese have known about this sort of energy influence for a long time. Louis Moss, M.D., one of the American pioneers in acupuncture and author of several books on the subject, has commented, "Chinese traditional medicine and philosophy is based on the interpretation that all things, animate or inanimate, possess an inherent factor of energy. Man is made of matter. He also has life. Thus he has two sources of energy, the electrical energy which is generated as a result of the biochemical and physical changes in the cells, and the living energy that he has inherited from his birth."[3]

The scientific community has long since accepted the idea of various force fields (electrical, magnetic, nuclear) and has recognized their existence and function in nature. By picking up certain energy patterns, bees find their way back to the hive, birds head north or south with unerring accuracy, monarch butterflies travel thousands of miles to lay their eggs. We humans must be subject to the exact same forces. If the energy exists for other animal species, it must exist for us.

And, of course, we create a lot of the energy on our own. Telephone relay stations, signals from the growing fleet of satellites, police radar, CB radios, and garage door openers—this is just the beginning of the list. TV screens give off their own energy, so do the video display terminals that tie the bank and supermarket to the main computer. Then there are burglar alarms and chickens roasting swiftly in microwave ovens.

The notion that the human body has an electrical component dates back at least to Galvani, and probably long before that. As you recall, Galvani, in his now-classic experiment, made the legs of a dead frog twitch by applying an electric current to them. These days, the correlation between electricity and the human body is pretty well established, but it was a startling revelation at that time.

If you have ever had an EKG taken to chart the action and condition of your heart, you know that the impulses recorded as squiggly lines on that narrow tape are the direct record of electrical currents generated by your own body. The same applies to brain waves and many other physical functions.

Dr. Burr, in one of his experiments to investigate electrical body fields, discovered that his instruments could measure the manner and speed of a broken bone's healing process. He has also had remarkable success in pinpointing the presence of cancer in women long before other clinical test methods could establish the fact. In both of these areas alterations in body force fields were utilized to gather the data.

We tend to think of ourselves as separate and distinct from the rest of the world and its forces. This, of course, is not so. In one of his lectures Alan Watts spoke of the human body as a bag of skin, within which most people feel enveloped and thereby separated from the rest of the world. In fact, the reverse is true. It is our skin that joins us to the rest of the world. We are part of it and of all of its forces; the electrical charges that are conducted by the surface of our skin are probably generated by and in turn regenerate the electrical forces all about us.

The electronic forces are new, but the idea is not. Hippocrates, regarded as the Father of Medicine, dwelt on the unity of man with nature over two thousand years ago. He believed that there is a vital force within man responsible for keeping the body in harmony. If something interferes with that force, disease is the result.

Within the past few years, additional credence has been given to the idea of body electric-force fields as the result of a procedure developed in the Soviet Union and now practiced in every country in the world, including the United States. The procedure is called Kirlian photography. In essence, it is the technique of photographing auras, the energy fields that surround and envelop the body. In the process, some hazy concepts previously regarded as unprovable have been firmly established. Demonstrating the existence of the acupuncture meridians is just one application of Kirlian photography. These force lines that guide Chinese medicine and medical philosophy are real. We can take pictures of them.

Other experiments have proven the existence of these forces, even though we may not fully understand them. For example, there is a biological test that has been repeated in many laboratories. A living cell culture is divided into two portions. Each half is put into a separate quartz test tube and sealed. The test tubes are brought into close proximity with each other, but they do not touch. Then the cell culture in one test tube is killed deliberately. Almost immediately, the cell culture in the other test tube dies. Obviously, some energy is transmitted via the quartz from one test tube to the other. The dying cell culture either kills off the other one or tells it to die. Someday we will understand what happens; for now it can serve only as a demonstration that natural forces do exist beyond our ken.

As you may have already surmised, this book will be introducing you to some powerful energies. Do not be alarmed. It is not nearly so exotic as it might seem at first glance. For indeed, we are surrounded by many apparently minor influences that can produce monumental results, but they are, by and large, phenomena as familiar as a simple magnet. As you probably know, when metal is magnetized, the molecules of which it is made are rearranged in an orderly fashion so that they are aligned with the magnetic polarity of the earth. Magnetism involves a major change—an alteration at the molecular level—and yet an intrusion of the slightest sort can effect this profound change. If you were to take a bar of steel and hold it aligned in a north-south direction and then were to tap one end of it with a hammer, the steel would become a magnet. You could prove it with a compass; you could pick up pins with your homemade magnet. Merely by tapping a piece of steel with an everyday household hammer, you could actually alter its molecular structure.

This is a very common thing in nature. Plants twist, turn, and contort themselves to face the light. That's their response to a force you can hardly feel. Vines grow in a spiral fashion, corkscrewing in one direction north of the equator and in the opposite direction south of the equator. Clearly, there is some elemental force at work here, yet for us humans, the only effect we notice when we travel from the northern to southern hemisphere is likely to be a slight hangover from the shipboard party that celebrated the event.

In the measurement of energy and specifically of body force fields, MRT acts as a very specialized type of indicator. In one respect, it's like the needle on an electric meter, which points to a precise reading. At the same time, MRT resembles a scale that tells either how much has been ladled out or how much more is needed to reach a preset weight.

Let's examine the scale analogy further, because understanding how this type of measurement works is essential to understanding MRT. Basically, there are two types of scales. One is the kind commonly used to weigh food. For example, you want to buy a pound of coffee beans. The store is a pretty fancy establishment and the coffee beans are in large bins. To fill your order for one pound, the clerk dips into the container and pours the beans onto the pan on the scale.

He starts with one scoopful and the scale reads four ounces. Another scoopful brings the scale up to nine ounces. It may take a couple more scoops to reach the one pound mark. All along the way, the pointer has been edging upward. Bit by bit, it has recorded the increased weight as scoop after scoop of beans is dumped onto the pan.

The other kind of scale operates in a different fashion. Instruments of this type are used in pharmacies, laboratories, and other settings in which precision is required. To work this kind of scale, you set it for the weight you want to reach. If you were weighing coffee beans on it, the first scoopful of coffee would not register at all. Neither would there be any movement of the pointer when you added the second or third scoops of coffee. But when you dumped in the fourth scoopful, you would exceed the preset one pound weight. Then, and only then, would the balance shift. The pointer would thunk over to the other side of the dial.

The amount that provided such a dramatic difference was, in itself, quite small, but the change that it indicated was enormous.

This is a fairly familiar set of circumstances in many phases of medicine. If you have ever had a complete medical checkup, you may recall that the doctor examined your eyes very carefully. Among other things, he was searching for evidence of ruptured capillaries in the retinal tissue way in the back of your eyeball. In themselves, they are not overwhelmingly serious; they are, however, a valuable indicator that blood vessels elsewhere in your body may also be suffering the effects of atherosclerosis, which is a sign of big trouble. The capillaries are small, but as an indicator they are enormously important.

MRT is another such indicator. In terms of the pattern of your overall physical health, a muscle that loses or gains strength seems of minor significance. As an indicator of the larger health picture, it is of major significance indeed.

CHAPTER

FOUR

# Landmarks

The MRT procedure depends in large part upon making contact with specific spots on the body of whoever is being tested. The accuracy of the response depends upon your ability to pinpoint those spots with precision. The body points can, for the most part, be located with reference to prominent bones, hollows, notches, and bumps. These anatomical features, what we call *landmarks,* are your key to the precise location of the body points. As such, they are an essential tool in the MRT process.

Bear in mind, however, that the landmarks are intended to lead you to specific points, not general areas, so it is of utmost importance that you learn to use the landmarks correctly so you can isolate the test point precisely every time you do the MRT procedure.

Let's take some time to identify the various landmarks and run through the easiest way to find them. Follow along with the descriptions and illustrations, and practice until you can find on your own body the exact spot indicated. It will be your first step in becoming an effective MRT tester and a cooperative MRT testee.

### Collarbone (Clavicle)

Slide your hand down either side of your neck, until you meet the first bone on your trunk. This is your collarbone, and it has two sections, one on either side of your body. Notice that one end extends out to the shoulder while the other end meets up with a flat bone, the sternum or breastbone, in the center portion of your chest. The landmarks to remember are:

*Collarbone*
*Center portion*—where collarbone meets breastbone
*Ends of the collarbone*—where it meets the shoulders on either side

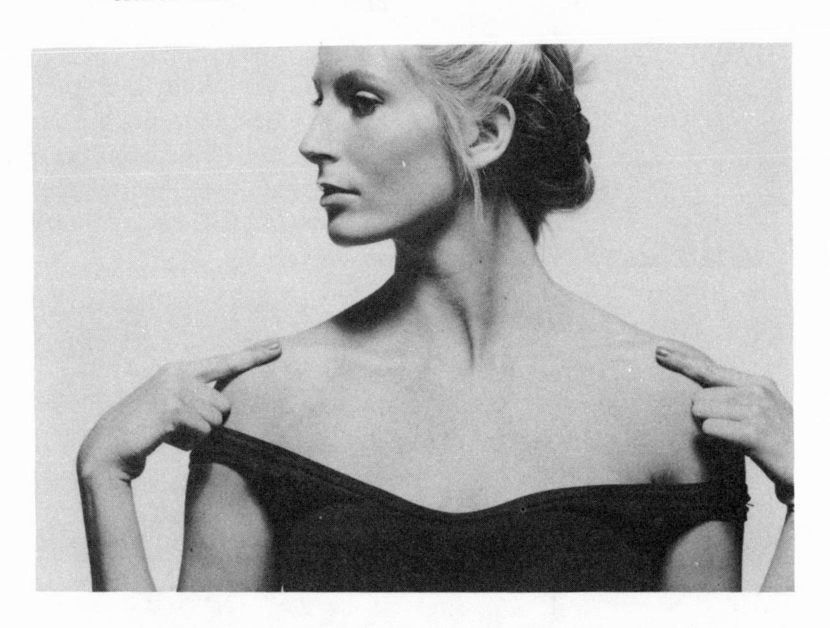

**Bony Notch of Collarbone**

Actually, this is a V-shaped notch in the top of the breastbone. Slide your fingers down the front of your neck past your Adam's apple. The first depression that you come to is the bony notch. It has two significant landmarks:

*The inner bottom point of the "V"*—some people have a bit of cartilage at this point. When locating a test point, ignore the

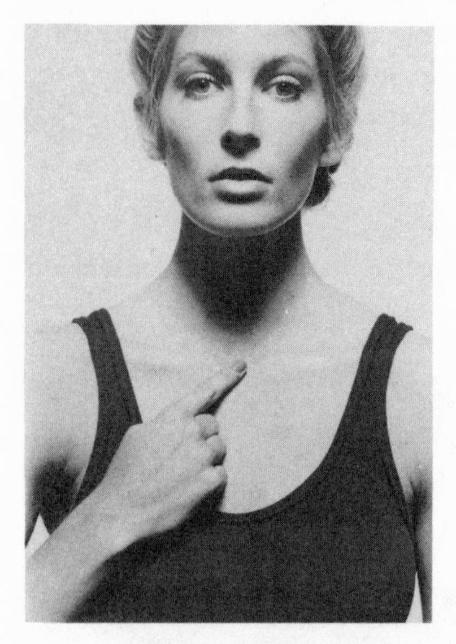

cartilage and take measurements from the bone at the inside base of the "V."

*The bony protuberances*—the two points at the upper edges of the "V."

**Jawbone Angle**

Place your fingers at the point of your chin and then slowly slide them along your jawbone until you come to a sharp angle just below your ear. That angle is the landmark we are seeking.

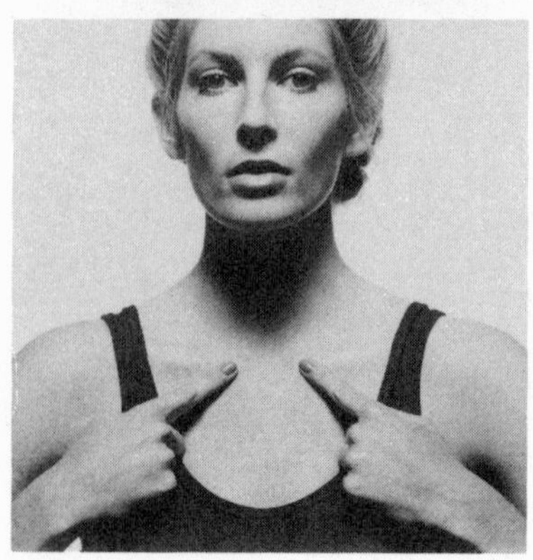

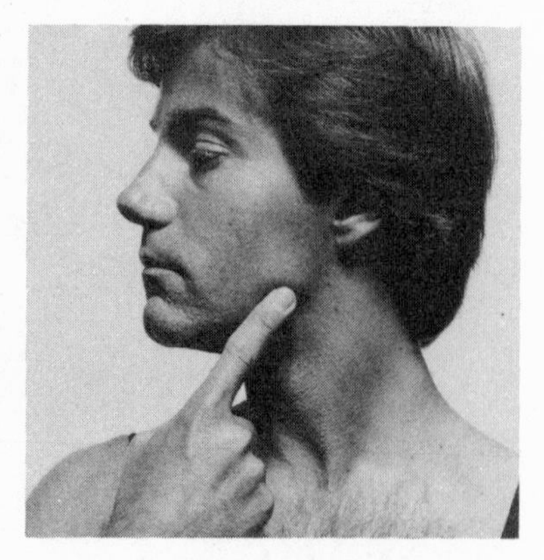

**Sterno Muscle (Sternocleidomastoid)**

This is one of the major muscles responsible for holding up your head. To locate it, place your fingers at the jawbone angle. Just below and in back of it, you will feel a rather sizable chunk of muscle. If you're not sure you've located the right muscle, move your head slightly from side to side. Follow the moving muscle downward until it meets your collarbone. Tip your head or rock it from side to side. The muscle whose course you have in this way followed is the sterno muscle.

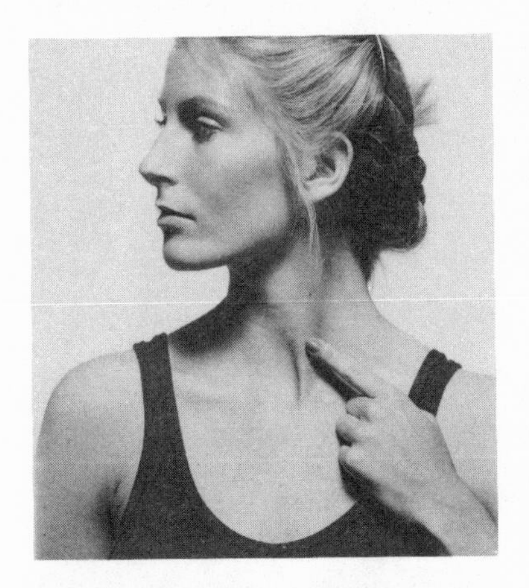

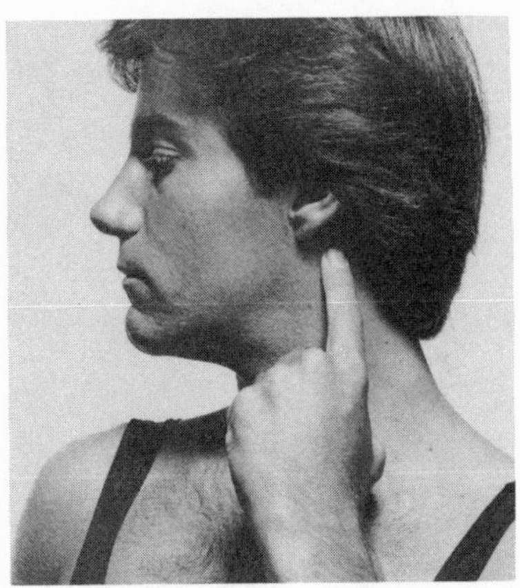

**Mastoid Bone**

Feel the back surface of your ear along the line where it joins your head. There's an arc-shaped bone on your skull at that point. It is called the *mastoid.* Run your fingers down that bone. At the point approximately level with the bottom of your ear, the mastoid bone comes to a point. This is the *point of the mastoid.* Do not confuse it with the hollow space below.

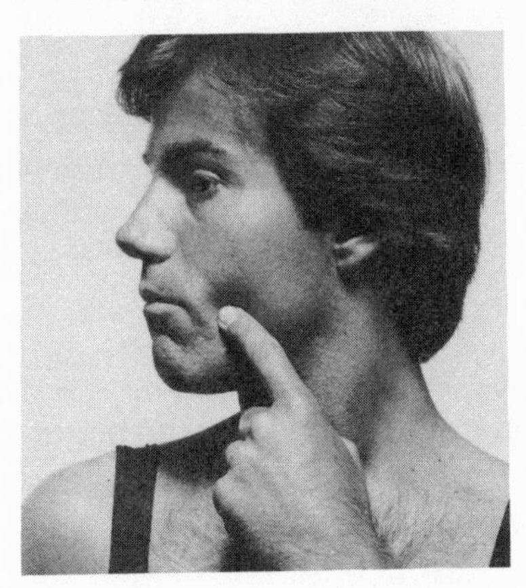

**Cheek Hollows**

Open your mouth slightly and suck in your cheeks. Poke a finger into the deepest portion of the hollow you have created, and you will be right on target.

**Frontal Protuberances**

Lightly rub your forehead. On a line up from each eye, midway between your eyebrows and hairline (or where it was in your youth), you will find two bony bumps. These are the frontal protuberances.

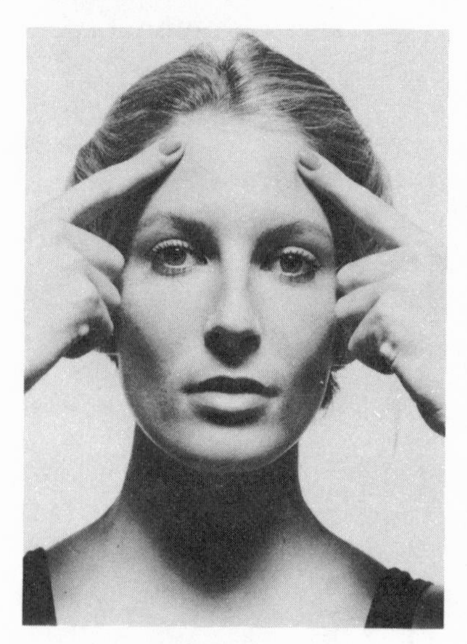

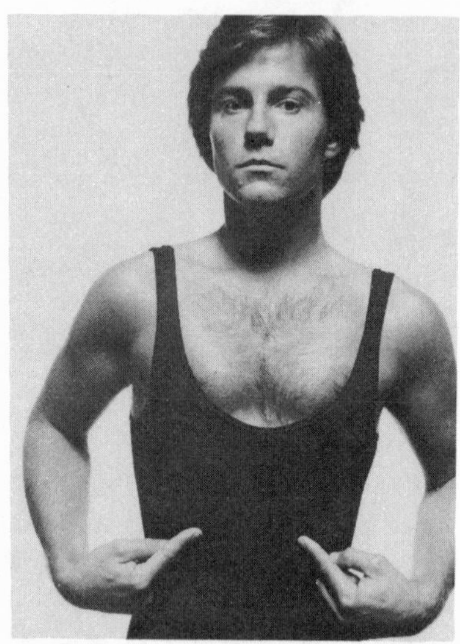

**Lower Border of Rib Cage**

Slide your hand down the front of your chest until you reach the bottom of your breast bone. Follow the margin of your ribs in a line extending from the center of your chest all the way around to your back. The course will be outward and downward, ending just above your waist.

**Lower Notch of Rib Cage**

You'll find this right in the center of your chest, at the bottom of your breastbone. Follow along the line just beneath the lowest rib, moving toward the center of your chest. At the exact mid-point, you'll find a notch much like that in the center of your collarbone, except that this one is positioned point up. Most men tend to have a little piece of cartilage fitted into place at the point of the "V" and projecting downward slightly. As a measuring point, use the "V" of the bony notch and ignore this cartilage.

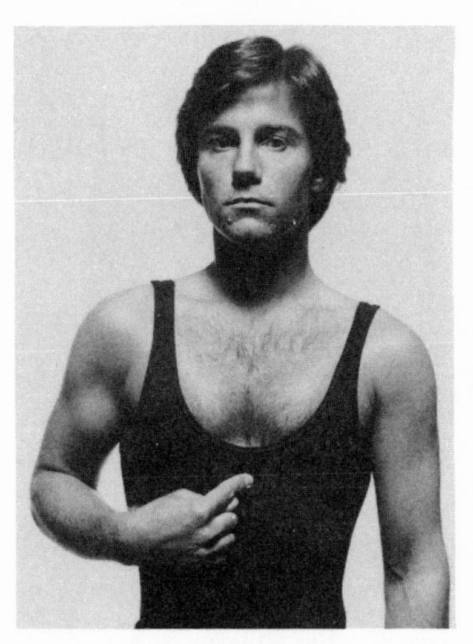

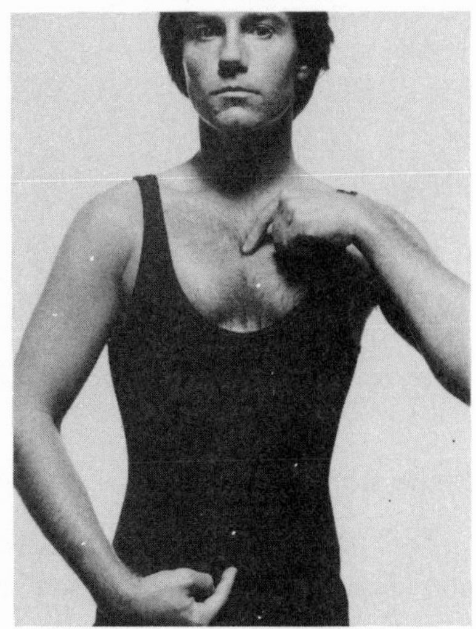

**Center Seam Line**

This is a vertical line that runs right down the center of your body in front. It divides your head, chest, and abdomen, passing through your navel.

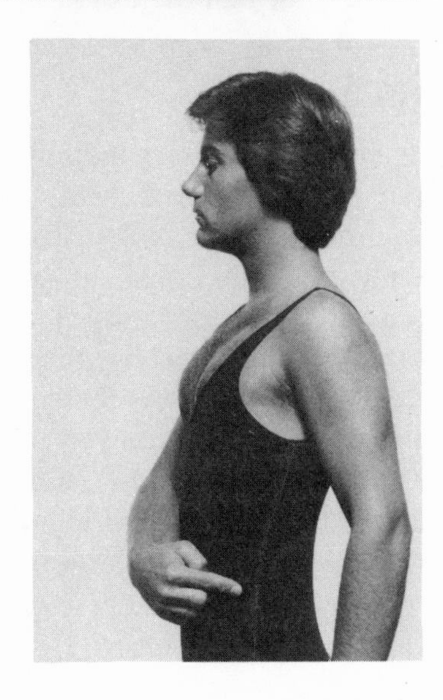

**Side Seam Line**

If your body were a shirt, this line would be where the seam of the fabric runs from under your arm and down the middle of your side.

**Stomach/Thigh Fold**

When you bend your knee and bring it upward, the crease formed between your thigh and your abdomen is emphasized. One end of this line is at your hip and the other just below your pubic bone.

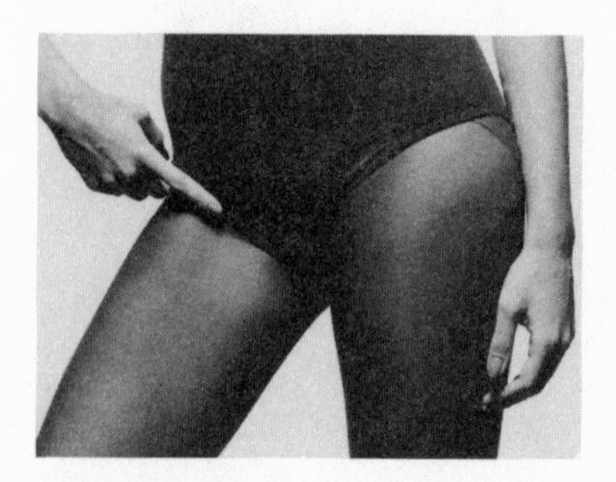

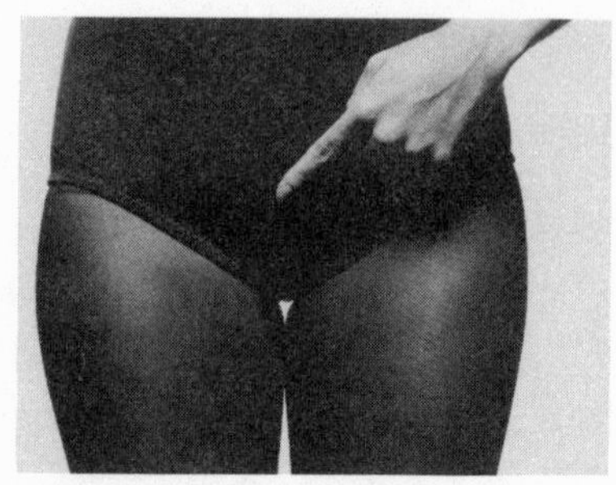

**Pubic Bone**

This bone is located in the lower portion of your abdomen, just above the genitals in both men and women. Press firmly until you have delineated the top or upper edge of this bone.

**Hip Bone**

Although the terminology is not strictly correct, what we call the hip bone is the part of the body that holds up your slacks. Our anatomical landmark is the projecting portion in the front of your body. If you are quite lean, you can spot this feature readily. If you are better padded, a little judicious prodding will reveal it.

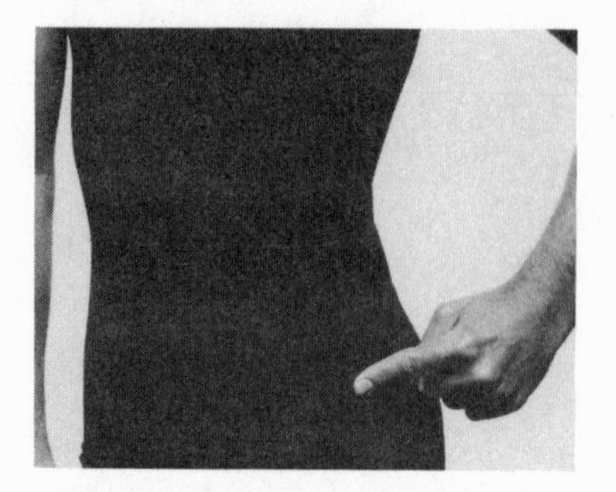

### Nipples

In males, this anatomical landmark is in a relatively standard position. The female figure, because of a great variation in the size and shape of breasts, presents a slight problem, for indeed it is not the nipple itself, but a point on the body located with reference to the nipple that we want to pinpoint. For the purpose of the MRT procedure, women should use as landmarks the approximate position their nipples would be in if their upper body proportions were those of a man.

### Last or Bottom Rib

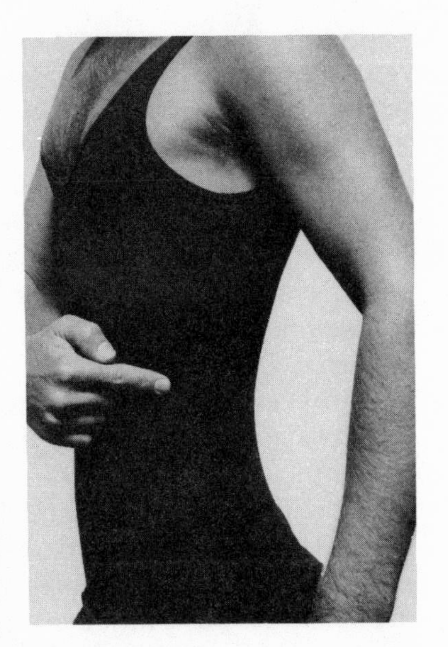

Starting under your arm, slide your hand downward, pressing as you go, until you have located the lowest rib. The exact position is slightly in back of the side seam line.

These landmarks will be referred to again and again in the course of this book. Because they play such a signal role in the MRT procedure, we suggest that you practice locating them and review them from time to time. Should you need to refresh your memory or take advantage of a visual aid, the descriptions and photographs in this chapter are here for that purpose.

CHAPTER

FIVE

# Vitamins, Minerals and MRT

If you have been even half awake for the past several years, you cannot have failed to notice that vitamins and minerals, those little-understood, much-talked-about components of the daily diet, have taken over center stage in the views of most people concerned about health and vitality. Vitamins and minerals have been held responsible for miracle cures of assorted maladies and crusades against such factors as aging, stress, overweight, and failing eyesight, to name just a few. In many ways, advances in the understanding of how vitamins work and what roles they play in human health and nutrition are enormously exciting. But to many of us, the whole field seems like a latter-day Tower of Babel. Confusion reigns, and the well-meaning, health-conscious consumer stands helpless in the midst of all the clamor.

One of the things that is most difficult about the whole matter is that whatever one might be able to learn about vitamins and minerals in general—anything from daily requirements and optimum dosages to contributary factors dictating special supplemental needs—is of little practical use to any one individual. A vitamin program, to be truly safe and effective, must be tailored to individual needs. That makes sense, but it also sounds like it costs a lot of money. For how can one get that sort of individualized prescription without resorting to extensive and expensive lab tests and expert diagnoses. The answer is MRT. Because MRT uses your body as its laboratory, it is possible for you to use it to design a personal nutrition program.

Before we look at the specifics of how MRT can accomplish this seemingly miraculous feat, let's get an overview of the whole business by listening to what some of the saner voices in the nutrition debate have to say about vitamins and the American diet as it now stands.

The U.S. government summed it up pretty well in one of its recent yearbooks.

"Food contributes to physical, mental and emotional health. Food nourishes our bodies . . . people always have known they must eat to live—children to grow normally, and adults to keep strong. But food can do more than satisfy physiological hunger and carry psychological and social values. Modern science shows that all of us, regardless of purse, can add years to our life and life to our years if we apply knowledge about nutrition to our selection and use of food. Brain and nerve are nourished by the same bloodstream that builds brawn and bone. Persons of every age and in every occupation require food of kinds and amounts that enable their bodies to maintain the best possible internal environment for all of the cells and tissues."

Those are fine-sounding words, but how do they stack up against the realities? Another government publication makes this observation: "Many studies indicate that many families do not have diets considered best for the maintenance of good health and physical well-being." "Principles of Good Nutrition," also prepared by Uncle Sam, says that "many people still consume diets poor in essential food elements." The text goes on to say "but poor or borderline diets are likely to result in retarded growth and development, bad teeth, increased susceptibility to illness, and a constant sense of fatigue.

"Improvement of the diets of American adults will come when more of them realize than do now that some changes in our patterns of eating are needed." Behind that cautious officialese is a simple statement: Optimum health requires, among other possible factors, completely balanced nutrition.

Sad to say, few of us even approach the optimum. As Dr. H. Curtis Wood, Jr., put it: "Most Americans, even though they think they eat well-balanced meals, are actually lacking in certain elements, and would benefit from a good vitamin and mineral food supplement."[4]

Or listen to the words of Dr. Roger J. Williams, director of the Clayton Foundation Biochemical Institute at the University of Texas and one of the most highly respected researchers and pioneers in the field of nutritional therapy. "It is my viewpoint that each individual has a substantial responsibility for ordering his own life, including his consumption of food. If each will take advantage of the unity of nature, diversify his food, avoid too much refined food, cultivate body wisdom, and use nutritional supplements when informed judgment so dictates, I'm sure that better health will be the reward."[5]

Fine, but from a practical standpoint, what chance is there for the average person to approach this ideal? Quite frankly, not much. As Dr. Williams bluntly states it: "How do people get perfect nutrition—every item in just the right amount? The answer is, they don't. People get along on imperfect nutrition, just as corn plants growing in a field and producing ten bushels per acre instead of two hundred bushels, which is possible. A perfect food environment is as rare as a perfect climatic environment. In a perfect climatic environment, the temperature day and night, the humidity, the rainfall, the wind and the sunshine would always be right."

Even though proper nutrition seems like an impossible dream, it's essential that we continue to push toward it. The closer we can come to improving our nutritional intake, the better we will feel and the longer we will live. But shouldn't it be possible to get all the vitamins and minerals one needs just by eating the proper foods? Yes, of course, it should be. But that's an ideal situation; in fact, we don't eat that way at all. If you doubt this, just read the label on a pressurized container of whipped topping (you'll notice they don't even call it whipped cream) or a jar of coffee lightener (again not a word about cream). Or if you'd like an exercise in pure terror, read the fine print on the side of the package of those chocolate-dipped cupcakes that are sold in the corner candy store and dispensed by automatic snack machines. Chances are you'll be halfway through the list of ingredients before you hit anything that sounds even vaguely edible. In some instances, not one single item contained in that cellophone-packaged treat has ever had intimate contact with the earth or a living creature.

This is how we squander one of the most vital paths we have toward achieving decent health. Dr. E. Cheraskin and Dr. W. M. Ringsdorf, Jr. say:

"We are convinced that every disease, physical and mental, is generated by a combination of circumstances which arise both inside and outside the body. It logically follows that disease may be prevented or cured by correcting variables that exist both inside and outside the body: We can go after 'germ' but we can also correct the life condition which predisposes the individual to illness."[6]

One of the most important of those "life conditions" is food. Which brings us full circle, and back to the question of how on earth one is to know what and how much one's body needs, at any given time, and how best to obtain it.

Until MRT there was really no way except trial and error, even on a professional basis, to work out a precise schedule of nutritional supplements. Even ortho-molecular physicians, who specialize in the correlation between nutrition and health, had to conduct their investigations in a hit-or-miss manner. Employing a procedure they call fine tuning, they first work out the *approximate* quantities of various vitamins and minerals their patient should be taking. Then they schedule a series of return office visits to check how well the patient is responding and to adjust the dosage accordingly.

But aren't there routine medical tests—analyses that can be performed in laboratories—to determine nutritional needs? Yes, there are. Trouble is, most of them are extremely complex and more than a few are quite expensive. For example, your doctor can order tests to determine the levels of iron, calcium, phosphorus, $B_{12}$, and folic acid in your body chemistry. Except for the test for iron, which is a fast and inexpensive one, the rest of this routine could cost a bundle of money. And then what do you have in the way of results? You find out the *level* of the specific element, but you learn nothing about your individual *need.*

Before MRT, a lay person who tried to determine personal nutritional needs on his own was engaging in an exercise in futility, a complete guessing game. Even now, most people resort to reading books and magazine articles on vitamins in general and then try to match up the symptoms they experience with the particular supplement that is supposed to correct this problem.

For example, let's say you have a persistent skin irritation, or maybe white spots on your nails. Practically every chart in existence says these problems are caused by zinc deficiency. The trouble is not every case of skin irritation can be corrected or even alleviated by zinc. The same goes for white spots on the nails. They simply are not always a sign of zinc deficiency.

Another example: Let's say that you have noticed that minor injuries don't seem to heal very swiftly. In other words, if you scrape or abrade yourself, it seems to take longer than you think is normal for the condition to finally get better. So what's advised? Vitamin E. What does this buy you? Do you actually get better? Perhaps. In some cases, stepping up your intake of Vitamin E can significantly shorten the time that it takes your body to heal. But there are other instances when it will make no difference whatsoever. The problem can be caused by some factor other than a shortage of Vitamin E.

As a matter of fact, by shifting your nutritional input, you may be responsible for causing a problem. Vitamin E is not a water-soluble material; it is fat soluble. That means that excess quantities are stored rather than excreted by the body. In this respect, Vitamin E is considerably different from Vitamin C.

You have undoubtedly heard a great deal about the supposed beneficial effects of large doses of Vitamin C. Presumably, you have also heard that there is no danger of overdosage because the excess will be simply eliminated by your body via your urine. In general, that's true, and it is because Vitamin C is water soluble. The oil- or fat-soluble vitamins, on the other hand, can build up to a toxic level in the body.

One more example. Let's say that you have been having some trouble lately getting to sleep. All the "experts" say that increased calcium intake will prove to be very soothing. Is this so?

Again the answer is an unqualified "yes and no." Yes, under some circumstances, calcium, taken in moderately large doses toward the end of the day, can have a soothing effect that will make getting to sleep easier. At the same time, the body that has trouble sleeping is the same body that may, without its owner knowing it, have a problem caused by build-up of calcium in the kidneys. The last thing in the world that body wants is more calcium, which will exacerbate a potential kidney stone problem. Better to find some other method of wooing sleep.

And we've just been talking about physical complaints, frank symptoms of deficiency. What about plugging up nutritional gaps before they start to cause problems so great that they alter the picture of your general health? As far as we know, there is no method besides MRT that provides an answer to that question.

And even if you have managed to ascertain, to a degree that makes you feel secure, which vitamins you need, there remains the question of how much of each you should take. That's when the self-prescriber begins to find himself stuck knee-deep in the dosage controversy. The first thing you will probably run across is an alphabet soup in which are floating such combinations as MDR and RDA, with little footnotes marked "na," "ne," or when the going gets really tough, a string of asterisks. (For the curious, MDR is the abbreviation for an old-fashioned term, *Minimum Daily Requirement,* which has been supplanted by RDA, which means *Recommended Daily Allowance, Required Dietary Allowance* or some other variant, depending on who is doing the talking. "Na" and "ne" are the old standbys, *not applicable* and *none established,* which get used whenever one approaches a realm in which little is known and less understood.

And then there are megadoses, a concept that has created something of a nutritional stir recently. Some doctors maintain it is the only way to achieve proper balance and good health. Accordingly, they recommend massive doses of some supplements in proportions that may be hundreds of times the standard dose.

The opposite of this approach also has its stalwarts. In this instance, minute amounts of vitamins and minerals are prescribed, the theory being that the body should be encouraged to foster the mechanisms that utilize specific nutrients.

But you can take a sidelines approach to this entire question. Theories, initials, formulas, balances—none of it matters when you use MRT.

With MRT, your body is the laboratory. And it's also your own computer, giving an instant and accurate readout on the supplements you need, plus the exact amount you should be taking of each. And that is the secret of any effective nutritional program. Unless it is designed for you and keyed to your individual, specific needs, it's a shotgun approach with all the hit-or-miss odds that implies. The point we're making is this: The selection and use of vitamin and mineral supplements should not, under any circumstances, be haphazard. Despite the easy availability of the materials themselves, this is no game for amateurs. It is in this precise area that MRT can make a fundamental difference.

Thanks to MRT, you have at your disposal for the first time a technique that will enable you to establish a meaningful correlation between the actual state of your health and the materials needed to bring it up to top level. Nutritional precision is now within your own reach.

CHAPTER

SIX

# Using MRT to Design A Personal Nutrition Program

It's probably clear to you by now that we think MRT is a pretty fabulous tool for anyone engaged in the quest for good health. In the area of personal nutrition, it has a very specific application, which we will explore in depth in the pages that follow. But before we get into the testing procedure itself and how best to utilize it, it's a good idea for you to fix a personal goal firmly in your own mind.

Okay, you say you are striving for good health. But how do you define that? What does that mean in terms of the way you arrange your life? The requirements of your own life-style? The limitations or ambitions you set for yourself? After all, a sense of well-being is just that—a *sense*—which means that it is a relative thing that has meaning for the person who experiences it. And that is you.

Maybe we can help you put this in perspective. Here's a checklist of easy-to-spot, easy-to-evaluate physical signposts you can use to evaluate your present state of physical well-being as well as your outlook on life.

1. Do you enjoy good sleep? Is it relatively uninterrupted? Do you awaken refreshed?
2. Do you feel energetic? This is a quality no instrument can measure, but if you do feel energy, you will be aware of it.
3. In your own evaluation, would you say that your mental outlook is good? Do you look forward to upcoming events? Do you anticipate pleasure? Do you, for the most part, take delight in living from day to day?

4. Do you enjoy food in moderate amounts? Can you readily distinguish between good food and bad? This doesn't mean you have to be a certified gourmet, rather that you are aware of what you're eating and whether you are deriving pleasure from it.
5. Except for odd occasions, are you relatively free from constipation and/or diarrhea?
6. Would you say that you rarely have headaches?
7. Except for occasions when you might make contact with something like poison ivy, is it unusual for you to itch anywhere on your body?
8. Are you spared a relatively constant assortment of aches and pains—of the back, joints, etc.? Does your body move easily and freely without any apparent stiffness?
9. Do you only rarely suffer from what you might call abnormal tiredness? We mean by this the sort of fatigue experienced when you haven't really done enough physical work to warrant exhaustion and yet you feel exhausted.
10. Are you relatively free of mood swings? Would you say that most of your emotional life is on a relatively even keel?
11. Is abdominal distress a rare event in your life? Is it unusual for you to experience gas or heartburn or do you constantly munch on antacid tablets?
12. Within a few pounds, is your weight relatively normal according to insurance-company charts? Are you not more than five to seven pounds either overweight or underweight?
13. In your own evaluation, would you say you enjoy life? This includes all of its facets: work, play, love, relationships with others. For the most part, do you find living fun?
14. Do you have a sense that everything in your life "works," both physically and emotionally? Obviously, you're not a machine and there will be some days that are better than others, but by and large, do things move along nicely in your life?
15. If someone were to ask you how you feel, could you most of the time state, "I feel great"? And do you really feel great? This is a conclusion that only you can reach. It involves a zest for life and living that manifests itself in an overall sense of well-being. Do you qualify?

The "yes" side of these questions is part and parcel of a healthy nutritional balance. The negative side suggests the need for a carefully designed program of vitamin and mineral supplements to provide the elements your body cannot produce (or cannot produce in sufficient quantities) from the food that you take in, either because your diet is lacking in the elements you need or because a malfunction within your body prevents it from utilizing the food you eat. A properly applied MRT program will enable you to identify and fill in the deficiencies, to measure and correct the imbalances.

There is an essential point we would like you to keep in mind as we embark on this quest for nutritional balance. Vitamins and minerals are not intended to "treat" any illness, imbalance, or other deficient body condition. They are not a medicine. The basic premise of nutritional therapy is far more subtle than that. Unlike the sledgehammer effect common with chemical medicine, vitamins and minerals encourage the body to respond. The correction of any condition comes from your own body. Vitamin and mineral supplements serve only to give it a nudge in the right direction.

As a matter of fact, we are convinced, along with many leading doctors and nutritionists, that tablet supplements are not even the best way of accomplishing this. (Remember, *supplement* means something added to fill in a gap; it does not mean primary factor.) A far better approach would be to get the nutritional boost you need from food sources. Unfortunately, this is difficult, and sometimes impossible, today. Foods are routinely "fortified," "enriched," or "nutritionally boosted," which sounds better than it actually is. Anyone who reads the fine print knows that these are euphemistic ways of saying that the nutritional elements inherent in the ingredients were removed or destroyed in the manufacturing process and a portion of some of these elements returned to it, although generally in chemical form. "Enrichment" on these terms truly leaves us with the short end of the stick. This is why so many people have to turn to vitamin and mineral supplements in tablet form. In planning your personal nutritional program, however, we urge you to try, wherever possible, to make food your primary source of vitamins and minerals, reserving tablets for the supplementary role when you need help in making up the balance.

And finally, may we remind you that it is always a wise idea to check with your family doctor before making a radical change in your diet. This is particularly relevant if you plan to increase significantly the dosage of vitamin and mineral supplements you will be taking. As valid as megavitamin programs may be for many people, there could well be factors in your own physical makeup that make it wiser for you to follow a slower, less dramatic approach.

**The Testing Procedures**

The Muscle Response Testing procedure for vitamins and minerals works in a manner similar to the sample test you tried with the aspirin bottle back on page 15. The deltoid muscle of one arm is used as an indicator of the effect of a test factor; the muscle responds by retaining its baseline strength or by weakening.

There are actually two distinct parts to the design of a balanced nutritional program with MRT. The first part involves determining *which* vitamins and minerals you need; the second part will tell you *how much* of each is needed. Part one utilizes as test factors specific contact points on your body, each one corresponding to a particular nutritional substance. You undergo testing by touching the prescribed point while a friend gauges the relative strength of your deltoid muscle. If the muscle remains strong, your current diet provides you with sufficient levels of the element in question. If the muscle weakens, this is an indication that you need additional amounts of the substance. It's really quite simple, but the procedure must be followed precisely if you are to get an accurate response.

Let's examine in detail the steps involved. You may find it helpful to refer back to the *landmarks* we outlined in Chapter Four if you are at any time unsure of the location of a contact point on the body.

Two people are needed for the testing procedure: the subject—that is, the one whose state of nutritional health is being inquired into—and the tester, a friend to assist the subject in his inquiry by means of MRT. The instructions that follow will be addressed largely to the tester, since it is he who to a great extent directs the procedure, but remember that *tester* and *subject* are temporary roles which can be reversed. Once you have helped a friend determine what his vitamin and mineral needs are, attention can turn to your own nutritional requirements and the two of you can repeat the procedure. With MRT, turnabout is always fair play.

Begin by relaxing for five or ten minutes. Simply sit quietly and give yourselves a chance to unwind.

Both of you should get rid of all metal you might have on your persons. The list includes wristwatch, jewelry, fountain pen, keys, coins, pocket calculator, and metal belt buckles. Do not be concerned with minor bits of metal such as the eyelets of shoes. We are primarily focusing on metal that is in direct contact with the body or present in larger quantities.

The concern about eliminating metal from the test situation has some logic behind it. Because the testing uses the body's reactions to, and its involvement with, certain force fields, which are probably electric or magnetic in origin, it makes sense to eliminate any substance capable of conducting an electrical current or responding to magnetic force. In practical terms experience has shown that factors such as these can interfere with the absolute assurance of a valid reading.

It's also a good idea to eliminate synthetic fabrics from the test situation. The reason behind this is that some people are allergic to some synthetic fibers, and a weak muscle response might, in that circumstance, be to the allergen rather than to the vitamin or mineral being tested. If it is not practical to remove every shred of synthetic material, proceed anyway; the chances are good that the response will be pure in any event. If, however, you cannot get a strong response to anything, it is reasonable to suspect that there is an allergen of some sort present. Serious steps should be taken to identify that allergen and to eliminate it from the controlled test environment. (You will learn all about how to isolate allergens in Chapter Seven.)

## Getting Ready

The first preliminary step is always to neutralize the subject. Begin with a fifteen-second massage of the points one inch to the right and left of the center seam line directly below the collarbone. Using the tips of the three middle fingers of each hand (or the index and third finger of one hand) and a firm circular motion, press hard enough to move the skin and some of the underlying tissue, but not so hard as to cause any discomfort to your subject. The second massage point is at the tip of the mastoid bone behind each ear. Repeat the circular motion, again for fifteen or twenty seconds. Finish up by pressing and releasing the tips of the mastoids six times without lifting your fingers, applying three to five pounds of pressure. (Test your touch on a bathroom scale first if you're not sure how much this represents.)

The subject should now be neutralized. If you want to check on this, we explain how on page 71, in our discussion of special situations and special tests.

Incidentally, the neutralizing procedure may be useful in itself. There are any number of things we do in the course of our daily lives that have a tendency to interrupt our neutral balance. Restoring that neutral state can be enormously helpful in maintaining a sense of well-being. For example, if you have been driving for a long time, it may be worth your while to have a traveling companion neutralize you at regular intervals. Whenever you stop for a rest or cup of coffee, a quick massage of the neutralizing points will make you feel more alert, less tired, and better equipped to continue with the trip. Various other stressful situations can be met more easily if you stop from time to time to get neutralized.

## Testing to Determine Which Vitamins and Minerals You Need

The procedure proper begins with a test of the baseline strength of the subject's deltoid muscle. He should stand or sit in as relaxed a posture as is possible. This does not, however, include crossing his legs, an action that can interfere with the accuracy of the test readings. He raises one arm, holding it out to the side at an angle slightly greater than ninety degrees (wrist and hand a bit higher than shoulder). His elbow should be straight, his hand open and palm down. He should keep his other arm hanging loosely at his side without touching his body.

As tester, you press against the back of his raised wrist with your fingers, steadying his body by placing your other hand on his other shoulder. Exert only a couple of seconds of pressure on the raised wrist. Practice until you can apply the force smoothly. The idea is to gradually but swiftly increase the pressure to maximum and then ease up smoothly.

Do not test the muscle more than five or six times before calling for a rest period. If you tire the muscle, it is hard to get an absolutely clear reading. The aim is to have a muscle strong enough to provide a contrast with the weak response you may be eliciting. This becomes difficult with an arm that is tired and therefore weakened by fatigue. You can, if you like, switch to the other arm for a while, but you may both prefer to take a five-minute break before continuing. This is a cooperative venture, so check with each other along the way.

You should both also remember that MRT is not arm wrestling or anything vaguely resembling it. The measure of strength and weakness is relative and it exists within the test subject's body. It is a before-and-after sort of thing, not a test of wills. This attitude is important to establish early on, particularly if children or ill or elderly people are being tested. It is evidence of nothing at all if a vigorous, healthy adult can force down a child's arm. It is the tester's responsibility to be acutely aware of the *change* of strength, the alteration in the amount of force he must exert to make the arm move.

Once you have established baseline strength, part two of the test begins. The subject will now touch various points on his body, each one corresponding to a particular vitamin or mineral, while you test to see if the deltoid muscle weakens or remains strong. As tester, you should keep a record of those vitamins and minerals that give you a weak response. (The items on that list will be the substances for testing in segment two, the determination of *how much* of which nutrients the subject needs. Appendix II, *Vitamins and Minerals,* will fill you in on all the background you need about these nutrients.)

The subject should touch each test point with the three middle fingers of his hand. The proper position is none other than the Boy Scout sign—little finger is folded to the palm, the thumb pressed down over it; the other three fingers are extended. The contact is made with the fingertips and the touch can be light since no real pressure is necessary.

Test the deltoid muscle of the subject's arm after directing him to the desired contact point and making certain that he has located it correctly. If either of you is uncertain about the location of any point, refer back to the *landmarks* in Chapter Four and to the photos in this chapter. Remember not to tire the muscle; five or six items at a time is enough and a five-minute break should be taken before you continue testing.

We'd like to stop a minute to review and elaborate on this whole strong/weak response pattern we have been talking about. Most of the time, strength and weakness are relative concepts, vague and difficult to measure in any meaningful way. When you are practicing MRT these two words have a precise and clear meaning.

A strong muscle feels as if it has locked into place. It is not at all spongy feeling. Without applying undue force, you cannot move the arm down; in fact, when you release the pressure, the arm seems to spring up a bit.

A weak muscle gives way. It will do so quite suddenly. It isn't a matter of wearing down the physical strength of your subject. Instead, when you apply force to his arm, he may resist for an instant, but then his strength will be broken. It will feel as if he has given up. You can move his arm downward quite easily.

**Body Contact Points for Vitamin and Mineral Test***

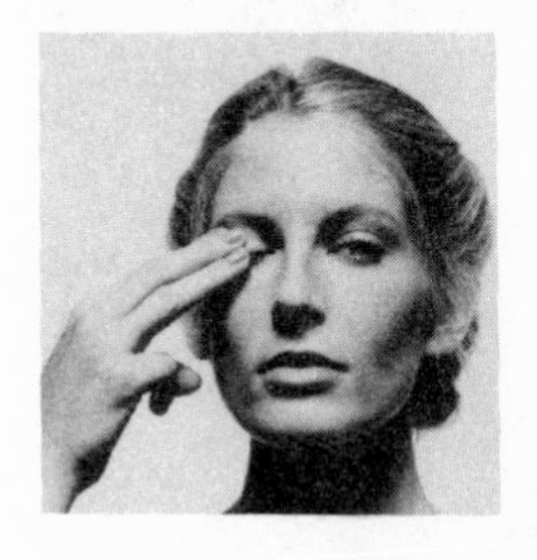
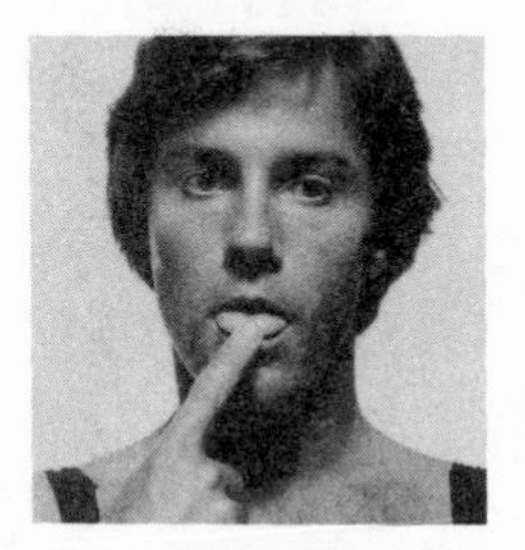
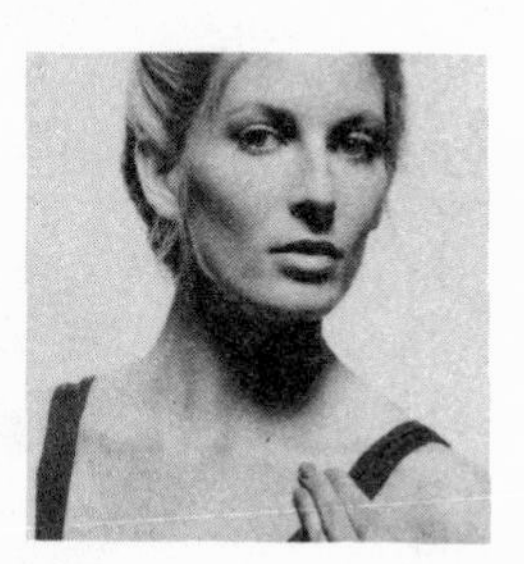

VITAMINS

*Vitamin A*: The right eyelid.
*Vitamin B Complex*: The tip of the tongue (also see note at the end of this listing).
*Vitamin C*: Just below the collarbone on the left side. 2½ inches from the center line.

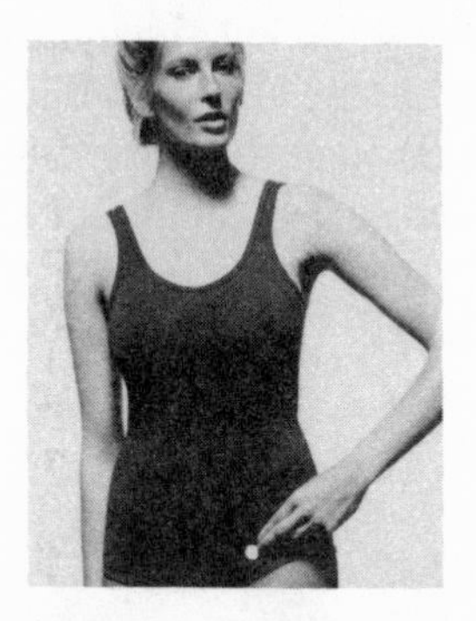
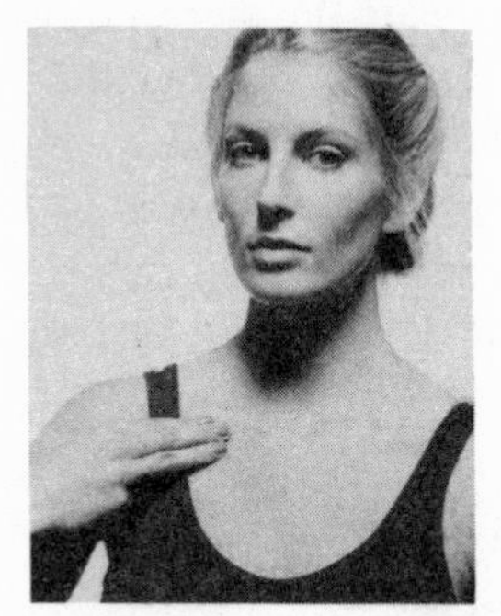

*Vitamin D*: Midway across the stomach-thigh fold on the left side of the body.
*Vitamin E*: Just below the collarbone on the right side. 2½ inches from the center line.

*The points and the procedure described in this chapter are an adaptation of basic techniques developed by Dr. Robert Ridler. He has given a series of seminars with instruction on a more complicated version of this concept geared to the professional, doctors who are interested in incorporating the method into their own practice. The procedure covered here is a scaled down version of the same approach intended for use by nonprofessionals.

*Vitamin F*: Locate the sterno muscle on the right side and slide your fingers down until you find the point at which muscle meets collarbone. Contact point is one-half inch above this.

*Vitamin K*: One-half inch to the left of the navel.

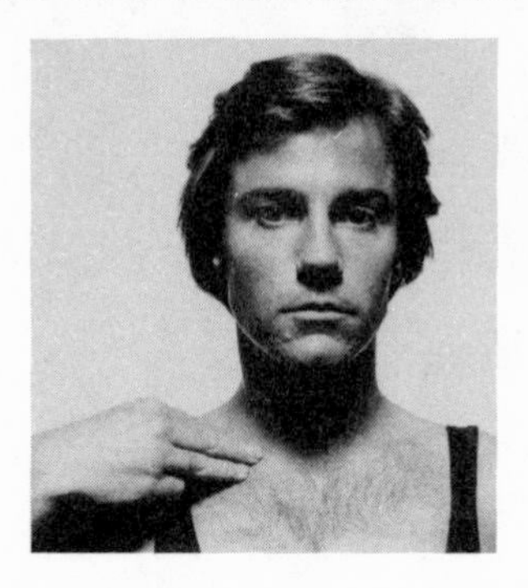

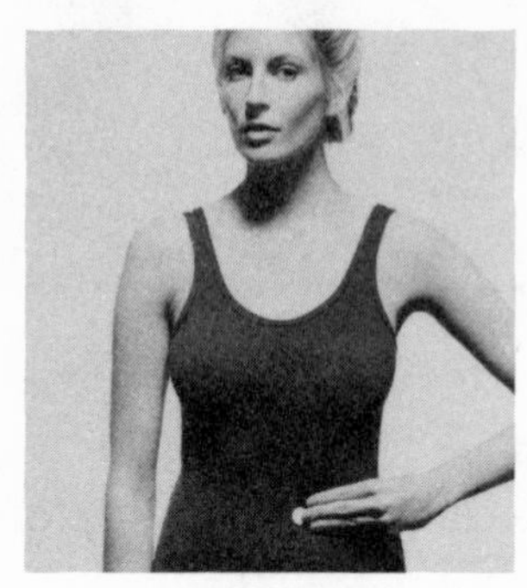

## MINERALS

*Calcium*: Locate the sterno muscle on the left side and slide your fingers down until you find the point at which muscle meets collarbone. Contact point is one-half inch above this. (See Vitamin F; this is the same location but on the other side of the body.)

*Iodine*: The soft portion inside the bony notch of the collarbone, just below the Adam's apple.

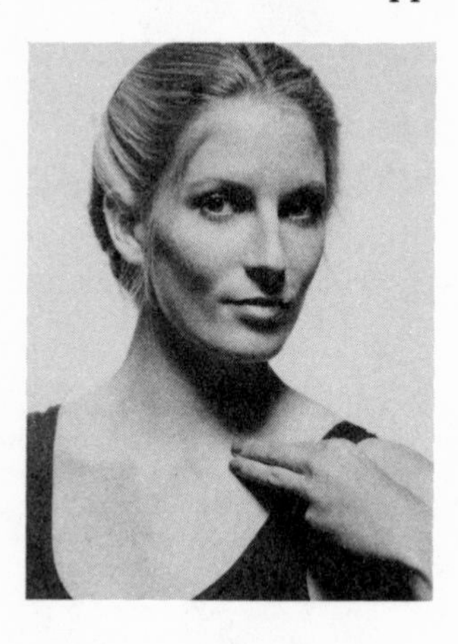

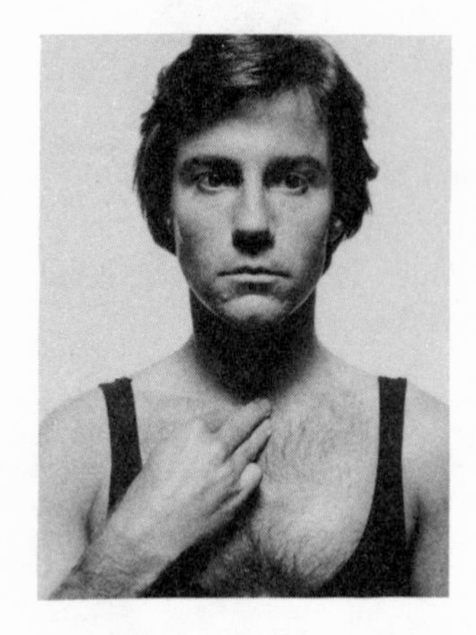

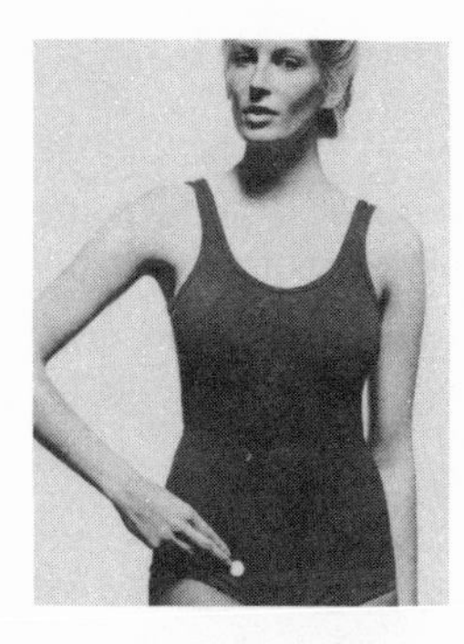

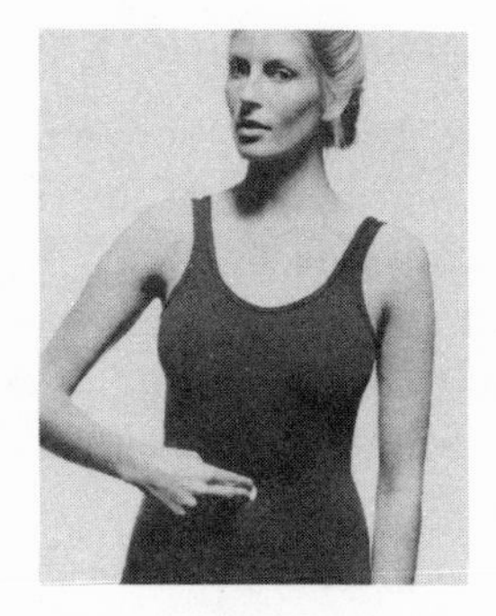

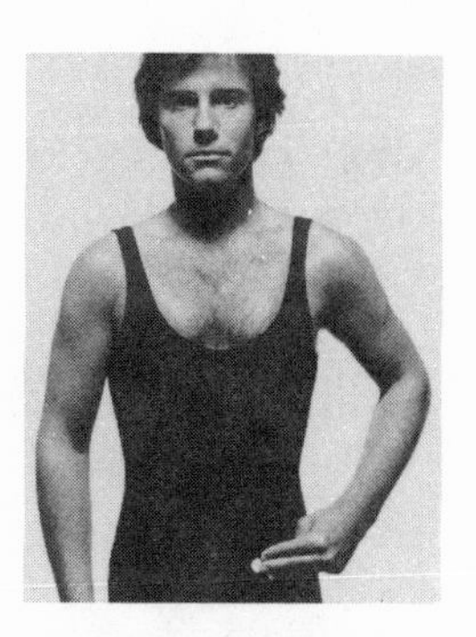

*Iron*: Midway across the stomach-thigh fold on the right side of the body. (See Vitamin D; this is the same location but on the opposite side of the body.)

*Magnesium and Manganese*: The middle of the navel. Note: To determine whether it is magnesium or manganese that is deficient, or if it is indeed both, follow the procedure for determining dosage detailed on page 55.

*Phosphorus*: Imagine a line running from the front of the left hip bone to the pubic bone. The contact point is midway between the two along that imaginary line.

*Potassium*: The hollow of the right cheek.

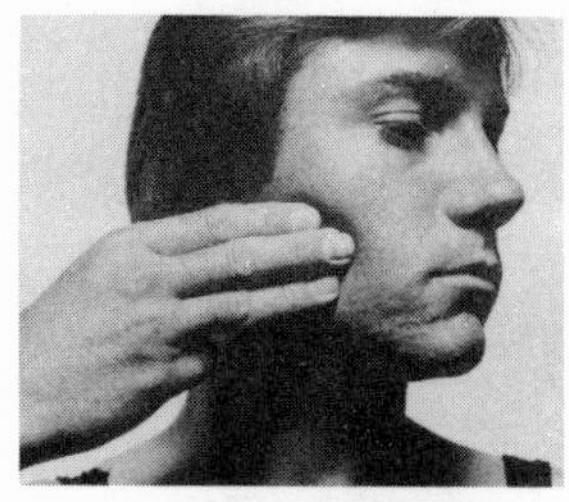

*Zinc*: Imagine a line running from the front of the right hip bone to the pubic bone. The contact point is midway along that imaginary line. (See phosphorus; this is the same location but on the opposite side of the body.)

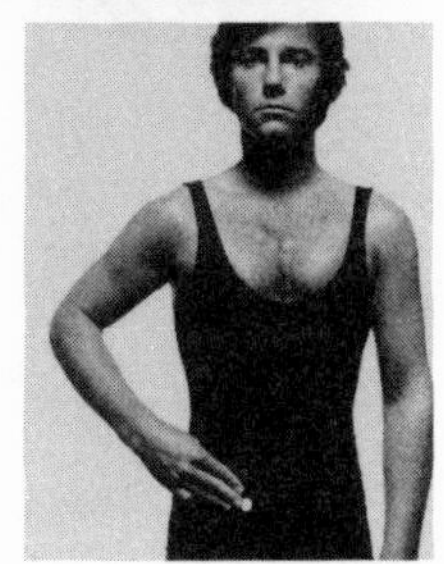

## OTHER NUTRITIONAL FACTORS

*RNA*: The bridge of the nose, just between the eyebrows.

*Enzymes*: Follow the lower border of the rib cage one inch to the right of the center seam line.

*Protein*: Grasp the hair and rub it firmly between the thumb and fingers, making certain that the hand does not touch the scalp. Obviously, the Boy Scout hand position is abandoned for this one.

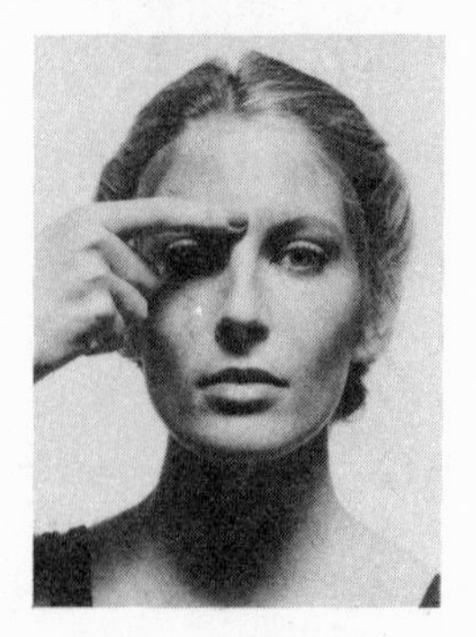

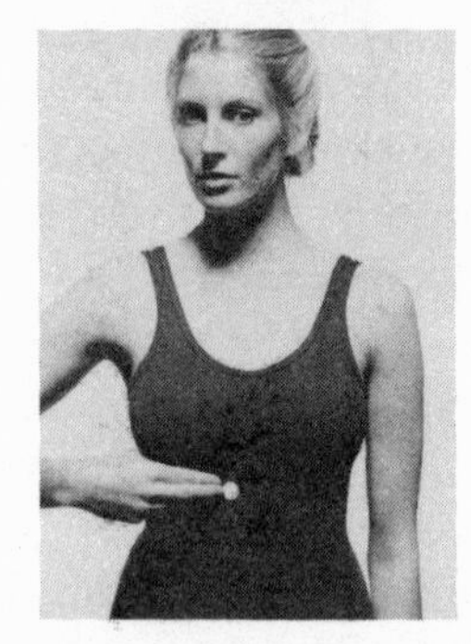

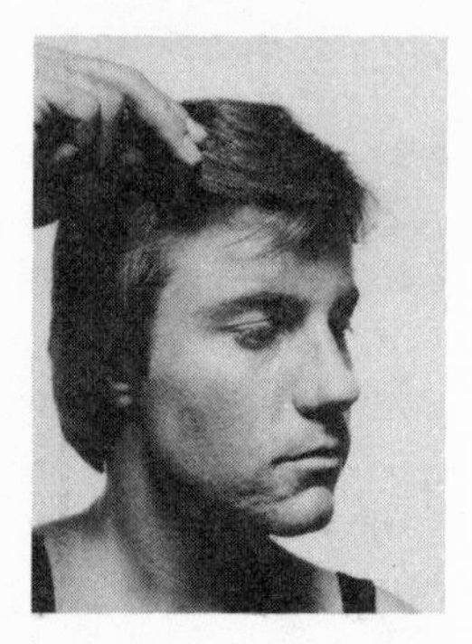

*Lecithin*: Two inches to the right of the center seam line level with the lower border of the rib cage.

*Hydrochloric Acid*: Follow the lower border of the rib cage one inch to the left of the center seam line.

*Thymus*: Two inches below the bottom of the bony notch of the collarbone along the center seam line.

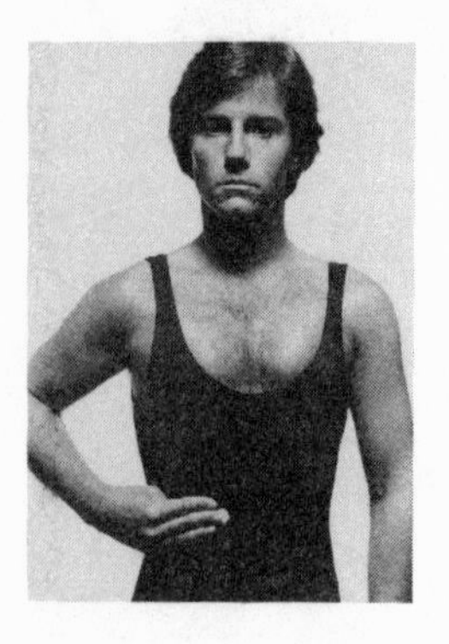

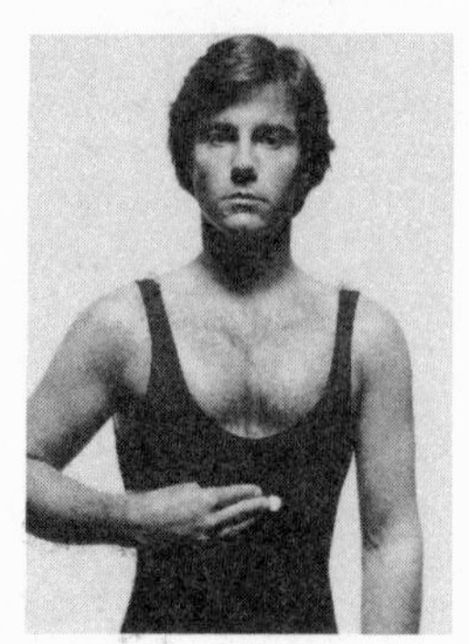

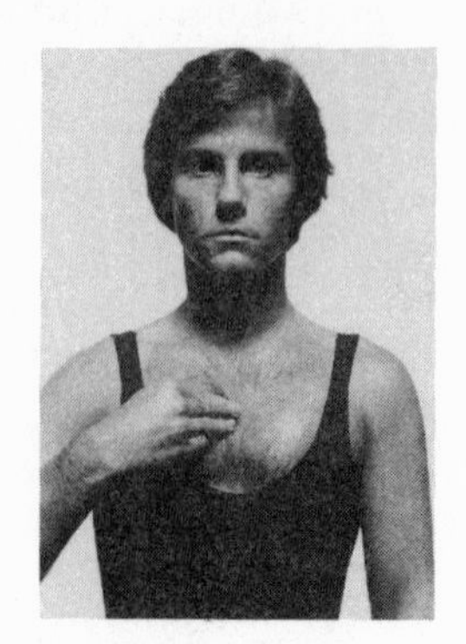

*Bioflavinoids*: Locate the outer edge of the bony protuberance of the collarbone on the left side. Trace a vertical line down from that spot to just below the collarbone.

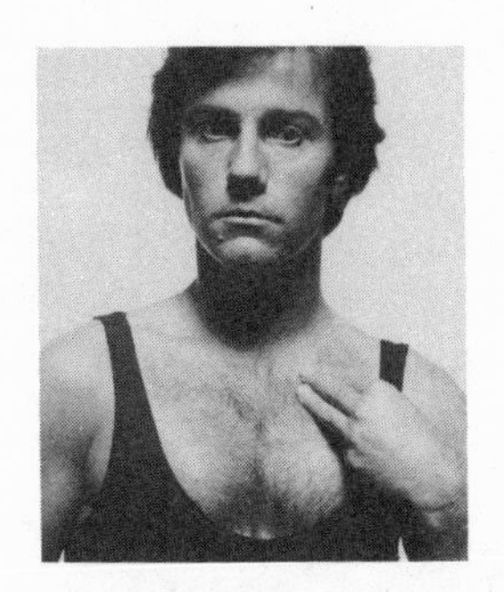

*Note*: If you wish to test for individual B vitamins (refer to the list in Appendix II) merely apply the dosage test. That way, you will be able to tell which of the specific components of this vitamin group you need (and how much), rather than lumping them all together and possibly taking more of one than is necessary simply because another in the group is called for.

### Testing to Determine the Dosage of Each Vitamin and Mineral You Need

Once you have figured out which nutritional elements you could benefit from in additional amounts, it's an easy matter to find out just how much of each you need. That's where the second procedure we spoke of comes in. Essentially, it's a variation on the basic MRT routine. You will need a companion to test you. In addition, you should have a bottle of tablets for each vitamin, mineral, and other nutritional factor on the list you ended up with after running through the first segment to determine *which* nutrients you need.

To get underway, follow the get-ready steps already detailed.

1. Both tester and subject should relax for a brief period of time.
2. All metal should be removed from pockets and persons of both participants.
3. Synthetic fabrics should be eliminated if at all convenient.
4. Tester should neutralize subject.
5. Tester and subject should assume proper positions, the sub-

ject standing or sitting in a relaxed posture, with legs *uncrossed* at all times and his hands are not touching his body.

The procedure involves having the subject make contact with each substance while the tester works the deltoid and observes the response. There are two ways to establish contact between the test tablets and the subject. He can hold them in his hand or he can place them in his mouth. The hand is, in several ways, preferable, at least for initial testing, since it keeps the tablets reusable. It is also possible that the dosage determined will be a rather large mouthful, though manageable as a handful.

You can do the testing on an ascending or descending basis. If you opt for the first alternative, the subject should hold one tablet of the nutrient being tested in his hand while the strength of the muscle of his other arm is tested. If it remains strong, up the quantity to two tablets. Continue adding tablets until the muscle weakens.

What is happening here? Very simply, when the muscle weakens you have hit the *toxic dose* of that material for the individual being tested. Reduce the dosage by one or two tablets and you will wind up with the maximum amount the subject can utilize safely in a program of dietary supplements.

Sometimes testing in descending order can save time. Take a guess at what you think might be the toxic dose and have the subject hold this amount in his hand. If his muscle remains strong, add pills one at a time until he does lose strength. Subtract two tablets and you have the maximum safe dosage. If the muscle tests weak immediately upon contact with this batch of pills, remove them one at a time until the muscle regains strength. Run through each item on the list you made, keeping track of the dosages you come up with. (You may also wish to test the individual B vitamins since this is, as we explained earlier, the best way to determine need and dosage of each member of the complex. Run separate tests for manganese and magnesium too.)

Be aware that this procedure is time-consuming and can be quite tiring to both subject and tester. Remember to take a break every once in a while. We think five or six muscle responses is as much as you should attempt between breaks. You may wish to do the tests over a period of several days. If you are in a really big hurry, or if you are encountering problems with the clarity of the response you are getting, check out Chapter Eight for some special tests for these special situations.

What you are looking for in each case is a strong muscle reaction. Too much will result in a weak response; the optimum dose will make the change to a strong response, whether you are working upward or downward.

But what happens if your muscle is always weak, no matter what is added or subtracted? This is a strong indication that you have an allergy to something involved in the test situation. Allergies to vitamins and minerals, in and of themselves, are rare, though certainly not unheard of. It is much more likely that you are allergic to the coating of the tablet or some other nonnutritional element in the particular formulation being tested. Try another brand and see whether that doesn't clear up the problem. We'll be talking more about allergies in the next chapter, for indeed, MRT can detect allergic reactions and track down allergens with the same degree of precision as it can determine nutritional needs.

A note of caution about mineral supplements. They do tend to have a cumulative effect; your body will excrete amounts in excess of what you need, but it does so very slowly. If you take very large amounts of mineral supplements, they may build up in your body faster than you can use or get rid of them. If the MRT test indicates that you are deficient in a particular mineral, it's best to add it gradually, working up to the dosage you have determined is needed over the course of several weeks. And do retest frequently during this period.

This is an area in which haste does not pay off. If it takes you even as long as two or three months to reach the optimum dosage, that is fine. Better safe than sorry, as they always say. Be prepared for some surprises; you may find in the course of one of your periodic rechecks that your muscle says "stop" long before you have reached the dosage it has previously told you was the ideal. Remember that MRT is a dynamic process that indicates what is going on in your body at the moment of testing. Test again another day. Since it is so simple to do the test, there is no excuse for not testing carefully and frequently. The payoff is your own improved health.

The testing process we have described can be one of the most valuable tools you have ever had at your disposal for obtaining and maintaining peak health. Remember, though, that what you will be doing when you follow the nutritional program you have designed with the help of MRT is beginning a healing and strengthening process which your body will continue. For this reason, it is essential that you retest periodically—we recommend every two months as a reasonable interval. You may be pleasantly surprised to discover that you need fewer supplements and smaller dosages of each as your body begins to renew itself and improve its utilization of the nutritional elements you acquire through your normal diet. It is also a good idea to recheck if you undergo a major change of any sort—for better or worse. For example, if you radically change your diet, if you have been ill or are suffering from a new physical complaint, if it is a time of unusual stress for you, if the circumstances of your life change in any significant way, test again and readjust your program accordingly. Because MRT can give you such a precise readout on your physical and emotional state, periodic retesting is a quick, easy, and accurate way to keep an eagle eye on your health and well-being.

CHAPTER
SEVEN

# Using MRT to Track Down Allergies

Tracking down an allergy is best tackled as a private investigation. For allergies are, by their very nature, intensely personal reactions, and in tracing the one that is deviling you, you will be traveling a path that is yours alone.

To be successful, you have to ferret out the particular substances that are poisons for you. And poisons they are, desite the fact that the culprits may turn out to be such basic foods as bread, coffee, doughnuts, or any of a host of ordinary fabrics or household items.

Allergic manifestations span the entire spectrum of human discomfort, from vague malaise and irritability to heart palpitations, violent skin rashes, and the terror of being unable to breathe. In most people's minds, however, an allergic reaction takes one course. You sneeze, your eyes run, and your nose becomes stuffed. True, this is a typical reaction; in fact, it's a classical one. But there are many other manifestations of allergy problems, and some of them may seem to you surprising, either because of their mildness or their bizarreness. For example, Dr. H. L. Newbold, one of the most highly regarded medical nutritionists practicing today, has observed a correlation between wheat allergy and schizophrenia. In his book *Mega-Nutrients* Dr. Newbold asserts that he has rarely tested a schizophrenic patient who was not allergic to wheat. Emotional problems triggered by food allergies are far more common, he claims, than most people realize. They do not always occur on the level of schizophrenia, of course; you may suffer less dramatic symptoms in the realm of mood alteration, but they too can be caused by allergy.

Allergies can be the demon behind pain in joints, a feeling so close to arthritis that you would be hard put to distinguish between them. Headaches are another common effect, ranging all the way from a low throb up to a full-fledged migraine.

If you've been feeling kind of down, if the zest for life that's been part of your emotional makeup seems to have dwindled, if you're not having much fun and nothing seems very satisfying, you may very well be in the throes of an emotional depression, but it could also be an allergic reaction. This sort of symptom is far more common than most people imagine. In place of mood-elevating drugs and intensive therapy (although both of these certainly have a legitimate role in the treatment of depression), tracking down and removing an allergic substance might produce an astounding cure.

Fatigue, the overpowering, constant sense of futile tiredness, is another direction that the symptoms of allergy can take. Ironically, that morning cup of coffee, plus a reinforcer for lunch and one or two more with dinner, can keep an allergy-prone person in a constant state of torpor.

Many and varied are the signs of allergies. It is possible to have a reaction to anything that you put in your mouth, even water. After all, it doesn't require any great stretch of the imagination to conceive of an allergy to chlorine, fluoride, or any of the other chemicals that are dumped into our water supply.

You don't even have to swallow in order to suffer an allergic reaction. Breathing will do it in some cases. You can be allergic to the inhaled particles of a perfume, of cigarette smoke. The skin is another entry point for allergens. Contact alone provides an almost endless series of possibilities. Allergies to fabrics are common. For the most part, these are associated with synthetic fibers (that's why we have been suggesting removal of these during the MRT test situation). It is, however, also possible to be allergic to such natural fibers as wool, silk, and cotton. Fur is certainly a frequent allergen. Dogs, cats, and even fur coats can be the culprits here. There are even cases on record of allergies to another human being—the skin, the excretions, the sperm.

In the attempt to isolate and identify allergic substances, you may have to shift your thinking a bit. In these days of miracle drugs and medical melodrama, we tend to look for extreme causes and violent reactions to qualify for blockbuster cures. This is not always the dimension within which allergies function. As elusive a feeling as being not quite up to par a good portion of the time can be a bona fide symptom of allergy.

From the standpoint of basic health, you should feel good all, or at least most, of the time. If you do not, the reason why bears investigation. You owe it to yourself to take the time, to take the chance to feel really good. For if you are successful in tracking down an allergy, the results are definitely worthwhile.

We guess what we are saying is that you should read this chapter even if you think you are not allergic to anything. Nothing bad will happen and maybe something good will.

Let's take a bit of time to learn about allergies in general. What are they really? What mechanism causes them? In very simple terms, an allergy is an overreaction by your body to the intrusion of an irritating substance. There are ways to be desensitized to the irritants, that is, to stop the body from reacting to the intrusion in such a hysterical way. But desensitization does not always work, and rarely is it 100 percent effective.

How about tests, then? Can't allergic substances be identified with clinical tests? Yes, they can, in some cases, but it means spending a good deal of time and even more money on what turns out to be a very fallible enterprise. That much-touted scratch test is so inefficient that many doctors have virtually abandoned its use. H. L. Newbold claims that the test is only 20 percent accurate in diagnosing food allergies. Those are pretty long odds when you are chasing something as elusive as a potential allergen.

And that brings us around to MRT. Unlike the less than impressive arsenal available until now in the battle against allergy,

MRT offers a highly efficient method of uncovering allergies. As with the tests to determine vitamin and mineral needs, the MRT allergy test has the power to give you a sure indication and positive proof. The procedure is a simple variation of basic MRT. Here's how to put it into effect.

The preliminary work is perhaps the trickiest. Essentially, you must design your own test population. Ironically, this is easier if you suffer from frank and dramatic allergic symptoms—you know when something has triggered your allergy alarm and you can begin narrowing down the possibilities. If you are at the other end of the spectrum—that is, if you are intrigued by the idea that your vague sense that all is not quite well could be an allergy and that you could attain a vigorous feeling of well-being simply by identifying and eliminating an allergic substance or substances—your task is more difficult.

Let's look first at the situation for the obvious sufferers. Begin by making a list of all of the foods you have eaten or substances you have contacted just prior to experiencing an allergic reaction. Most allergic reactions are fairly immediate, so generally there is no need to go back more than one day. It is essential, however, that you be extremely detailed and accurate.

For example, suppose that you ate, among other foods, a slice of apple pie. Merely to list apple pie doesn't begin to approach the problem. What was in that apple pie? The fruit, of course, plus sugar, pectin, cinnamon, lemon, and perhaps some other flavoring items. Was cornstarch used as a thickener? How about the crust? Flour, water, eggs, butter, salt, and what else?

The actual testing is done in stages. For the first, or gross, investigation, you use the various foods just as you ate them. For example, as a first line of inquiry, you *would* test apple pie. If it turned out that you were not allergic to it, there would be no need to test any of its individual components. If, on the other hand, the test indicated that you were allergic to the apple pie, you would then have to check out each ingredient that went into it to isolate the one that is causing your problem.

Bring in your test partner and go through the standard get-ready procedure, just as you would for any other MRT routine.

1. Relax together for five or ten minutes.
2. Remove all metal from your bodies, pockets of your clothes, etc.
3. Remove any clothing you might be wearing made with synthetic fibers (if it's convenient to do so).
4. Tester should neutralize subject.
5. Subject and tester assume test positions, making sure that the subject's posture is relaxed, and his hands are not touching his body, his legs uncrossed.

The test is conducted by having the subject make contact with the suspected allergen. It's like the aspirin routine you learned about at the start of all this. In this case, it's possible to hold the suspect (if it's a food) in the mouth, or if you prefer, to hold it against your body. Both methods work equally well.

If you do hold the food in your mouth, chew it for a few minutes, but don't swallow. The reaction that will be picked up from the MRT test is a sort of early warning. In effect, your mouth will be telling the rest of your body that there is a problem on the way. Your muscle strength will respond to this.

After testing each individual food, always spit it out and then brush your teeth and rinse your mouth thoroughly with water. Do not use toothpaste for this process. Wait two minutes for your reactions to normalize before you proceed with the next food.

Physical contact with the suspect food (or other substance) provides another effective test, and it may be more efficient. You can work with the material held in your hand, but for greater reliability, use as a contact point the bare skin two inches above your navel. Hold the food carefully so that your fingers don't contact your body.

There is a reason for this. As you learned in Chapter Three, the entire MRT process is primarily involved with readings of body force fields—body energies and the distortions of them. There have been many other discoveries that use this same general idea. Acupuncture, of course, is one. There is a very powerful acupuncture path, or meridian, located in a line from the midpoint of your skull all the way down the front of your body. It is known as the Vessel of Conception, and it corresponds to the landmark we have been calling the center seam line.

Another acupuncture channel, known as the Stomach Meridian, also passes through that same approximate area. This meridian is in the form of dual lines running parallel to the Vessel of Conception, and a couple of inches on either side of it. By placing the substance to be tested on this spot, you are bringing into play a very sensitive evaluation zone. It is, in effect, a leg-up on a more decisive MRT reaction. It makes good sense to use every advantage you can.

For contact testing of a food, first check to make certain you are not allergic to wax paper. In the rare event that you are, check out transparent plastic wrap. Place a small amount of the food, two tablespoons is about right (neatly wrapped in wax paper), against the test point on your stomach. Hold it firmly in place with one hand while your other arm is used for the test. A non-food substance can simply be held up to that spot. If it is wet or otherwise messy, it too should be wrapped in wax paper.

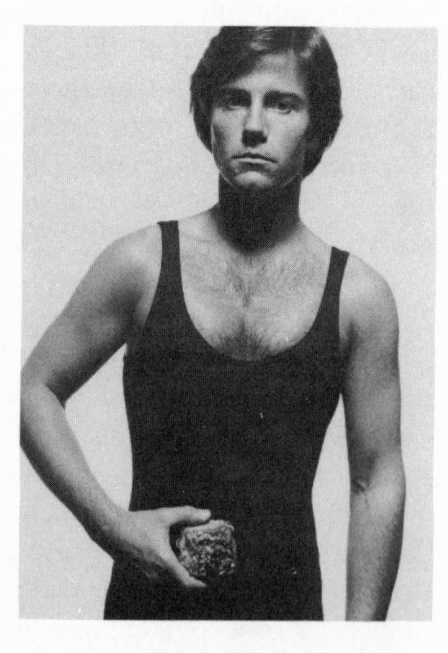

Test responses are to be read exactly as for any other MRT procedure. A baseline reading of your muscle strength comes first. Then you make contact with the test substance and retest. If you have no allergy to the substance being tested, your muscle will remain strong. If you do have an allergy to the material in question, your arm will instantly be weak. Again, there is no middle ground.

Subject any and all foods and other substances you suspect of being allergens to this test, taking care not to exceed the limits of the muscle's baseline strength by tiring it out. Take frequent rests whenever either of you feels tired.

Any investigator, but particularly those of you who are not certain if an allergy is at the bottom of your "down" feeling, should be aware of some conclusions from observation that doctors and nutritionists have made. Apparently, certain foods have a greater tendency to aggravate allergic reactions than others. This usual list of suspects is a good place to begin your investigation.

**Checklist of Common Allergy Producing Foods**

| | | |
|---|---|---|
| Apples | Eggs | Oranges |
| Bananas | Fish | Peanut Butter |
| Beans | Fruits | Salt (iodized, uniodized, and sea salt) |
| Bread | Grapefruit | Soft Drinks |
| Brewer's Yeast | Honey | Sugar |
| Butter | Hard Liquor | Tea |
| Cereal | Lettuce | Tomatoes |
| Cheddar Cheese | Mayonnaise | Tortillas |
| Chocolate | Meat | Vegetables |
| Coffee | Milk | Water |
| Corn | Oats | Wheat |
| Cottage Cheese | Oleomargarine | Wine |

You can expand the scope of your investigation and also zero in on possible allergic candidates by paying attention to food families. You see, there is an interrelationship between certain foods. The connecting thread is not always that obvious. The list that comprises Appendix III can be your guide.

For example, if it turns out that you are allergic to buckwheat, you should also check rhubarb and garden sorrel. Allergically speaking, there is a correlation between these, although taste, appearance, and all other factors may be totally different. Don't attempt to analyze this strange botanical fact. Just take it as gospel and use the list for your own advantage in your own test procedure.

There are two other elements that enter into allergic reactions to which you should be alerted. First is the frequency factor. Oddly enough, some foods do not produce allergic reactions each time they are consumed; some substances do not set off alarms each time you touch them. It is perfectly possible to get by if contact or consumption takes place at infrequent intervals. If the time span is shortened suddenly, you could wind up with an allergic reaction.

In other words, let's say the MRT procedure for allergies indicates that asparagus is a particular problem for you, yet you adore asparagus and have never had any difficulty with them. This may be because you eat asparagus infrequently and in modest quantities. If you were to step up the frequency—for example, celebrating the height of the asparagus season by eating them every other day—you might very well find yourself in the throes of a full-fledged allergic reaction.

Sometimes the amount of a specific food can be the triggering factor. You can get by with a little bit of ice cream, but should you dig into a double-scoop sundae, look out! Perhaps sugar doesn't ordinarily cause you problems, but in the course of one meal, you put sugar on your grapefruit, dumped sugar into your breakfast cereal, added sugar to your coffee, and then, for the hell of it, had an especially sweet piece of pastry. Trouble might come a-knocking.

Finally, food combinations can cause a very distinct allergic reaction even though each individual food that makes up that combination might produce no problems on its own. In other words, the group is toxic, but the individual elements are not. For this reason, you may be able to eat ground beef, pickles, bread or rolls, ketchup, and tomato as long as you ingest them separately. Combine them into a hamburger, and all hell breaks loose.

Obviously, the process of testing both complete food combinations and the individual ingredients will uncover any instances of this strange factor. We did want you to be aware of it, however, because some of your test results might otherwise appear to be totally devoid of logic.

You can extend the MRT procedure one step further and possibly avoid having to narrow your diet to a point you find intolerable. When you have finally tracked down the specific foods that cause allergic reactions in your own body, test them once more in combination with garlic pills or tablets. Many nutritionists believe that garlic can be a major factor in promoting digestion and preventing adverse reactions from foods singly and in combination. It's worth a try, and the process is not at all difficult.

To test, merely hold the offending food (wrapped in wax paper) against your body at the test point together with a few garlic tablets or capsules. If your arm weakens when you test without the garlic, but remains strong when you include the garlic capsules, the message is clear. Make a final test by eating the offending food along with a dose of garlic. Although it does not work for everyone, you may be lucky enough to have found a way to enjoy a full-range diet without problems.

Incidentally, most garlic pills, capsules, and tablets are compounded in such a manner that your breath will not become offensive, even when you have taken a great many of them.

The emphasis of the investigation we have been describing thus far seems to be on foods. Substances that come in contact with the skin can as effectively be tested with MRT, and you should search in those areas as well.

Be sure to make your individual selection from the list of objects that you actually contact during your normal routine. As a suggested starting point, the list might include:

Soaps and detergents
Deodorants
Ointments
Cosmetics
Hair sprays

The candidates do not end with personal products. After all, you are in contact with many more materials during your waking hours. The following is intended to get you thinking in the right direction. You can assemble a more complete directory by glancing about the rooms of your home:

Upholstery and carpets
Clothing
Fabrics
Leather shoes, handbags
Cookware
Pets

Clothing should be checked by using a representative of each group. For example, test one cotton shirt. If you are not allergic to cotton, you can cross all other cotton items off the list. Make sure, however, that they have no other fibers blended with cotton. You may be allergic to one of those. Be aware also that you can be allergic to the dye used for a particular garment.

The allergic potential of washable clothes can frequently be reduced or eliminated by adding a half cup of washing soda to each load of the automatic washer. This procedure is not 100 percent effective, but is at least worth a try.

Whether it is food, clothing, a cosmetic, a piece of jewelry, or even a favorite pet, substances that cause allergic reactions can be powerful, clandestine enemies to the allergy sufferer. Anyone who experiences trouble breathing, agonizing itching of the skin, or another in the broad range of allergic tortures should welcome this application of MRT. Others, who claim to be allergy free but who have vague complaints and minor, though annoying, responses to unknown factors in their environment, may also find that they can gain an improved state of general health once they have identified a heretofore unknown allergen and eliminated it from their lives.

For each of these groups of individuals, MRT offers an incredibly effective, inexpensive, at-home test that has it all over the traditional allergy scratch test and can offer us all lives free of the misery allergies can cause.

CHAPTER

EIGHT

# Special Situations and Special Tests

Nothing in life is one-hundred-percent predictable. This is especially true when you're dealing with human beings, with the human body and the human psyche. Since MRT is, at its very essence, a test of human response modified by human reaction, there is bound to be some variance.

Fortunately, the divergences and variations are within compensatable realms. The alternate techniques detailed in this chapter are intended to improve the clarity and firmness of MRT results should you encounter, as tester or testee, a test situation in which readings are a bit hazy. In general, the same procedural details apply to these specific situations as to the standard MRT process, except for the specific points noted. Be certain, therefore, to go through the neutralization and get-ready procedures and to conduct the testing itself in the same relaxed and quiet atmosphere as ever.

## Partial Response I

We have made the point several times in the preceding pages that the MRT response is unequivocal, that the muscle is either strong, or it is weak, and there is no in-between. In fact, you may, on very rare occasions, find yourself giving or getting a response that may not be as definitive as we have described. In this case, the tester should do a *temporal tap* around the testee's right ear only. The basis of this procedure will be examined thoroughly in Chapter Ten. For now, let us simply explain how to do it.

Before you attempt a temporal tap on someone else, follow these instructions to define the path of the tapping on your own head.

Begin just in front of your ear. Find the right spot by placing your fingers in the general vicinity and then wiggling your jaw. As you move your fingers slightly, you will arrive at a hollow just in front of your ear and about one third of the way down from the top of it. This is where you begin the tap; continue upward, about one-half inch from the ear, following a ridge of bone in the skull that pretty well duplicates the curve of your ear. Follow this bone all the way around to the back until you come to a rounded point—that's the mastoid bone and it is the end point of the tap.

To do the tap on someone else, use the three middle fingers of one hand and contact the head with the finger pads. Tap in a rapid series—about two beats to the second—in the arc described. When you come to the terminal point, lift your fingers and return to the front of the ear to begin again. This is a perfectly natural movement if you stand facing the subject and use your left hand. Temporal tap three or four times, then repeat the test procedure. This time around, the response should be far more definite.

**Partial Response II**

Dehydration can sometimes cause a response that is less than definitive. If you are having difficulty as tester in distinguishing between a strong and a weak muscle, ask your subject to drink a glass of water, wait a few moments, and then resume the test.

This is a relevant step to take if the subject has been engaged in strenuous exercise—if, for example, you are testing the efficacy of a jogging program and the subject has just done a sample run. Dehydration can also be caused by fever or an infection of some sort, so this factor is worth considering if the subject is ill.

**Tired Arm**

Let's suppose that, according to the rules of MRT, you have really done enough testing. The subject's arm is tired, and by all logic you should call it quits for a while. However, there are one or two more tests to perform and you would both like to finish up the session. In this case, the tester should place thumb and middle finger of one hand against the frontal protuberances on the subject's forehead, those bony bumps on a line running upward from each eye, halfway between eyebrow and hairline. Hold them there for thirty seconds, and then recheck the muscle's strength. In almost every instance, it will be strong again and will remain strong enough for one or two more tests.

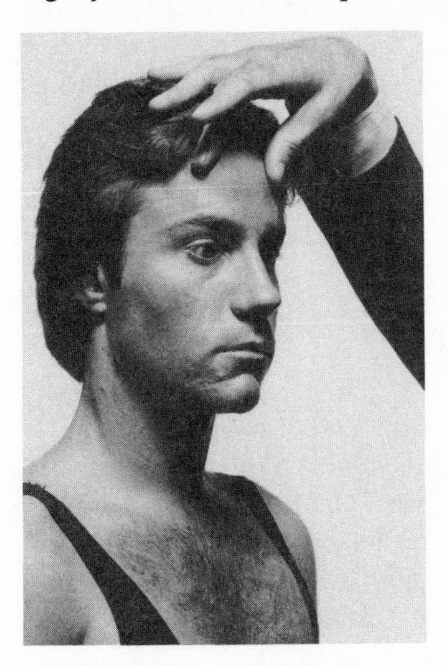

**Checking on Neutral State**

Every test situation must begin, of course, with the subject's being neutralized. But how can you be sure that the neutralization process worked or, having succeeded in neutralizing your subject, that in the course of a particularly lengthy or stressful testing session, nothing has occurred to disturb the neutral balance you have achieved?

In fact, there is an easy way to check your subject's neutral state. Make a determination of baseline strength in the usual manner: test the deltoid of one arm while your subject lets his other arm hang loosely at his side without touching his body. Next press your index finger into the cheek hollow on the side of his face opposite the arm you are testing. With your finger in position, test again. If the muscle tests weak, your subject has been effectively neutralized and remains so. If the arm tests strong—that is, if there is no noticeable change from the baseline test you made—your subject is not in a neutral state.

In the case of the latter, go through the neutralization procedure again, briefly massaging with the tips of your three middle fingers the points one inch out from the center seam line just below the collarbone and the point behind each ear at the end of the mastoid bone. After a fifteen-second massage at each of these locations, press firmly on each mastoid tip five or six times without lifting your fingers. Check for neutralization once again as described above.

## Stronger Vitamin Reaction

A simple way to intensify the MRT response when testing for vitamin or mineral needs is for the subject to wet his fingertips before touching them to the prescribed place on his body. Keep a glass of water handy for him to dunk his fingers into from time to time. The extra moisture will magnify the effect.

## Super-Strong Subject

Suppose you are in superb physical condition. You run, you do push-ups, sit-ups, and handstands; you swim and play tennis. In your spare time, you work out at the gym. Your body is so magnificently conditioned that it would take a diesel-powered winch to haul your arm down from a horizontal position. So how can anyone test you? If you cannot arrange to have King Kong do the procedure, simply ask your test-mate to weaken your arm.

A bit of background first. In traditional Chinese medicine, the acupuncture points that are used to treat various problems run in a series of meandering rows, called meridians, that snake their way across the body. If one of these meridians is stroked lightly starting from its initial point toward its end point, strength will be lost. Reverse the action by stroking from the end point in toward

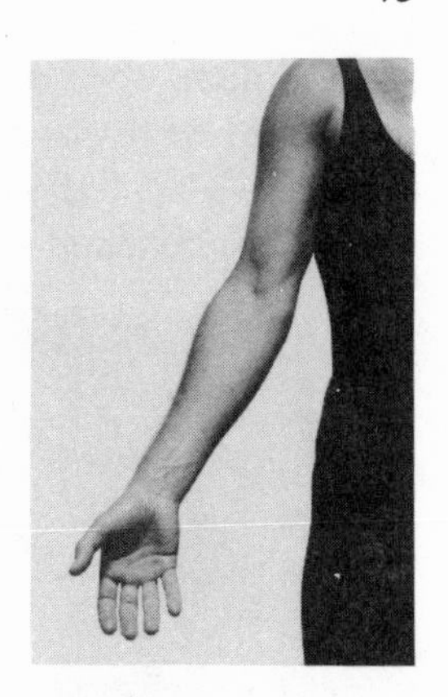

the beginning and strength will be gained. Perhaps the most convenient of these acupuncture channels is known as the Lung Meridian; it extends from the front of the shoulder down the inside of the arm and out to the thumb.

The person testing you should trace your Lung Meridian with his fingertips all the way out to the end of your thumb, four or five times. Each time he reaches the end he should lift his fingers from your body and move them back through the air up to your shoulder. You can then

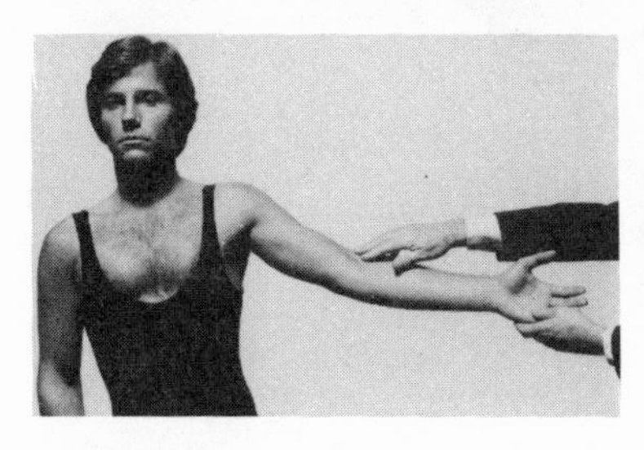

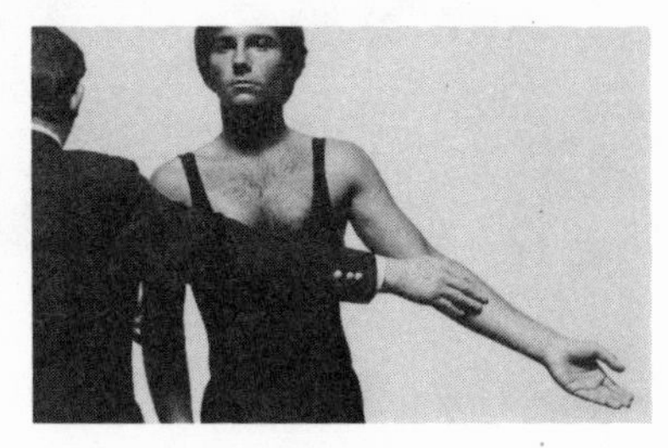

proceed with the test without your test-mate having to resort to superhuman force.

When the testing is finished, your full strength should be restored with a reverse stroke of the Lung Meridian, from thumb to shoulder, four or five times.

**Weak Subject**

Here's the reverse situation. In this case, the person who is being tested has so little natural strength that it's difficult for the tester to distinguish between the strong and weak response. The remedy here is to beef up the muscle strength.

The Lung Meridian is used, once again, but in reverse. The tester should begin at the underside of the thumb and trace with his fingertips and pathway up the inside of the arm to the front of the shoulder, four or five times as described above. A test will probably reveal enough strength in the subject to proceed. If not, the Lung Meridian should be traced a few more times until the muscle has reached a useful level of strength.

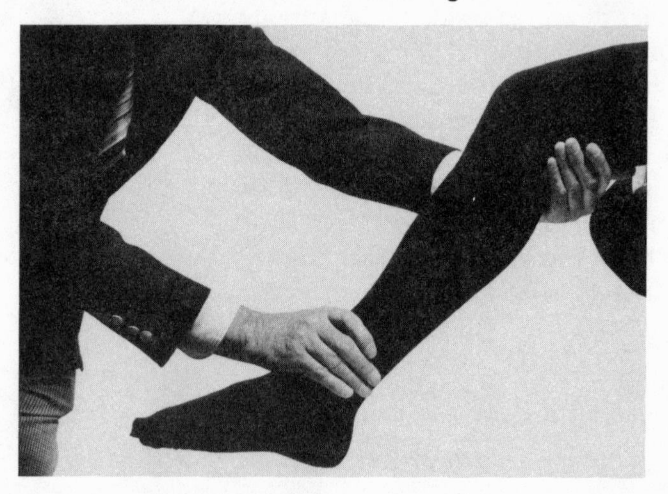

**Sitting-Down Test**

In various circumstances, it may be preferable to do MRT with the subject seated rather than standing. We have already stressed that this can be done, using the deltoid muscle, provided care is taken that the legs remain uncrossed. It so happens that you can also use a leg muscle as indicator, and in some cases this may be desirable. The muscle you use is called the quadriceps, the big muscle that runs along the front of the leg above the knee, what is commonly called the thigh muscle.

The subject sits with his leg outstretched until it is almost, but not quite, straight. The other leg should be bent at the knee but relaxed. Instead of holding the subject's shoulder with one hand to steady his body while you test, hold his upper thigh. Proceed as you normally would, deriving a baseline measurement of strength and then introducing the test condition and rechecking. The response is tested by pressing downward against his ankle with your other hand. If the muscle is weak, his knee will lose strength and bend easily. If it is strong, it will resist bending.

Keep this alternate procedure in mind if you ever have to do a test on someone (or yourself need to be tested) either with a cold or just recovering from one. The arm muscle used in the standard form of the MRT procedure is, according to classical Chinese acupuncture, connected with the lung. In fact, as you now know, the Lung Meridian runs directly through the deltoid muscle. For this reason, any physical disturbance that affects the lung (such as an upper respiratory infection) will tend to weaken the arm muscle, making a baseline measurement of strength unreliable. In such a case, you can frequently get a more valid reading by switching to the quadriceps muscle of the thigh.

### Testing Babies

Believe it or not, it is possible to effectively test a tiny baby, despite the communication and coordination difficulties inherent in the notion. Should a circumstance arise in which you want to test an infant, this is the procedure to follow.

You do need a third person, someone to hold the baby, and it seems desirable that that person be the child's mother or father. The tester need not be so closely related.

The parent should sit down and hold the child in his or her lap, being absolutely certain to sit with legs uncrossed. Because the parent acts as a conduit for the child's energies, the same caveat applies as when the seated subject is tested directly. The parent should make contact by holding one hand firmly against the baby's bare skin. The tester then proceeds with the normal MRT routine, using the strength of the parent's other arm as indicator. The response will be a perfectly valid reading for the baby.

Incidentally, although we have never tried it, we understand it is equally feasible to test a pet dog or cat in the same fashion. Presumably, you could determine what nutritional supplements would be beneficial to Fido or what foods might be troubling him with allergic reactions. But perhaps this is a demonstration better suited for inclusion among the "parlor games" we talk about in the back of the book.

**Hypoglycemia**

Although the standard MRT procedure is generally effective in detecting a negative response to sugar, another test is sometimes more accurate. For this procedure, the subject should stand with his fingers closed in a loose fist and his arm hanging straight against his side, thumb close to the body. The tester should try to pull the subject's arm away from his body while he resists. Note should be made of the baseline strength of the resistant arm. Next the subject places some sugar in his mouth—a sugar cube or a teaspoon of granulated sugar will do fine—and the test is repeated. If sugar presents a problem to the subject, his arm will be considerably weakened the second time around.

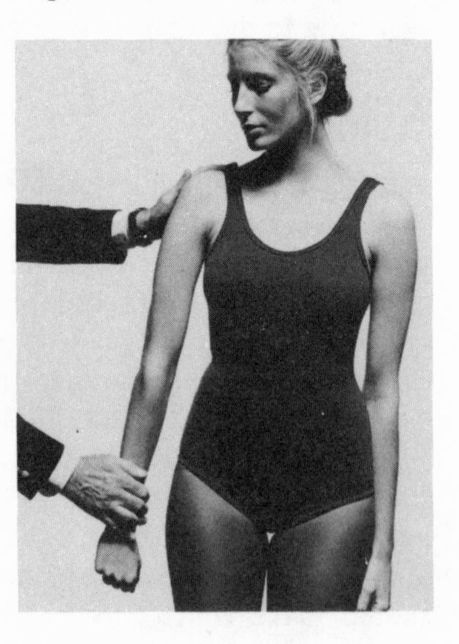

Note: If your response to this test is quite dramatic, we suggest you consult a medical doctor about the advisability of your undergoing a six-hour glucose tolerance test to confirm the possible existence of hypoglycemia.

**Unobtrusive Finger Test**

Upon occasion, you may want to check whether you are allergic to a specific food in a setting in which the full-scale MRT procedure would be awkward and embarrassing—in a crowded restaurant, for example. To avoid drawing a crowd, here's a substitute test that is remarkably sensitive as a detector of food allergies.

Press together the tips of your thumb and little finger on one hand. Your companion hooks one of his fingers under each of your two and tries to pull them apart while you resist. Do the test once before you have eaten anything to establish how much force is required to pull your fingers apart. Then put a tiny bite of the food in question in your mouth (do not swallow) and have your dinner partner recheck. In the presence of a food allergy, your fingers will lose a huge amount of strength. They will be unable to resist the force exerted by your friend. The difference between the strong and weak reactions will be sure and definite.

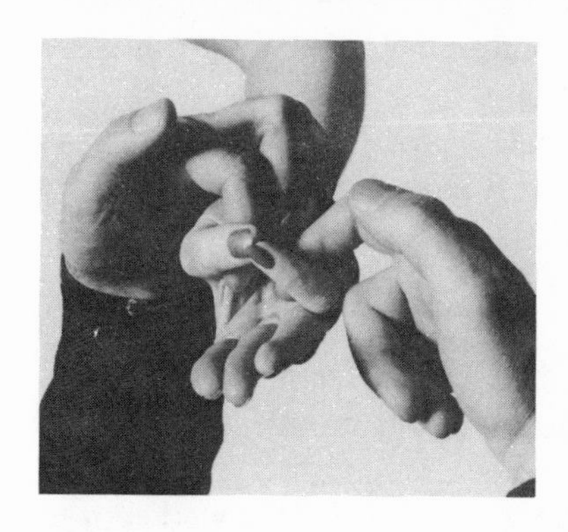

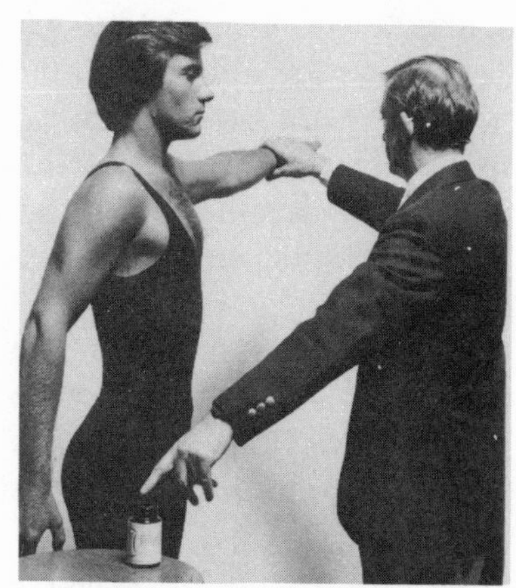

**Pointing Test**

This is an interesting variation on the MRT procedure which does not require the subject to make direct contact with the materials being tested. Although it will not work in all cases, if you have proven to be relatively sensitive to the testing routine, you may find that you will also respond to this method.

You do not hold or touch the substance for which you are being tested; rather, the tester merely points to it with his index finger while testing your muscle with his other arm. The index finger *must* be used, with all the other digits folded into a loose fist.

As we said, this system does not always work, but it *is* interesting and it can be useful when you are being tested for a great number of substances since it has the advantage of being faster than the standard method.

**Avoid This One**

There's an old story about the kid who was continually admonished by his parents not to put beans up his nose. In fact, it would never have occurred to him to indulge in this sort of bizarre behavior, but since his parents made such a to-do about it, he tried it to see what it was like. The beans stuck in his nose, of course, and a doctor had to get them out. We bring up this story because we are about to do the same.

There is one process that can bollox up almost all the test responses that immediately follow it. It makes the muscle virtually immune to becoming weak, at least for a short time. So. Here's something that in the interests of valid testing you should *never* do.

If you place your tongue behind your front teeth and then press upward with the tip against the roof of your mouth, your muscle will *not* weaken. Why? We don't know. It's another one of those happenings that must be investigated further before we begin to understand it. On a strictly empirical basis, however, it is known to turn test results all a-kilter.

CHAPTER

NINE

# Instant Emotional Therapy, With a Bonus

There is a kind of relief that MRT can bring to ease emotional turmoil or trauma. Please understand that this procedure is not, under any circumstances, a substitute for professional guidance or aid. It is strictly a short-term palliative that will temporarily smooth over some rough spots and soothe your nerves in some situations to some degree. It should not, therefore, be considered a cure for long-standing neurosis or deep-seated psychosis.

Within its own limits, however, this variation of MRT could be just what you need to help you get through a brief uncomfortable period or a spell of unhappiness. It differs, in this way, from the detection and correction of troubling thoughts we talked about in the last chapter. The emphasis here is on relief of distress, not modification of behavior or attitudes.

As before, the deltoid muscle is tested for its response to certain stimuli. In this case, a strong or weak answer reflects your emotional state. Perhaps you are skeptical about how this could be so. By now, the direct correlation between emotional distress and physical manifestations is an accepted concept in most schools of psychotherapy. We know that many migraine headaches have at their roots fear, anxiety, worry, or some similar emotion. We know that stomach distress is not always attributable to physical causes, that emotions can trigger intestinal spasms and increase the secretion of irritating stomach acid. The field of psychosomatic and psychoactive disease is very broad, and this particular MRT variant is just one more implementation of the body/mind connection.

Once again, a companion is needed to conduct the procedure. It is certainly a good idea to choose as your collaborator someone with whom you have a trusting and compassionate relationship.

Begin with the standard get-ready process, giving particular attention to the preliminary relaxation period. Once you have done this, removed metal, and been neutralized, place your thumbed middle finger of one hand over the frontal protuberances, those bony prominences on your forehead. While you do so, try to concentrate on the problem that is disturbing you.

You need not say anything aloud. If you like, you can indicate to your friend the general area of your concern, but this is by no means necessary. In this sense, you have all the privacy you require. Do be sure, however, to put all other thoughts out of your mind and to concentrate fully on the cause of your distress. Two minutes of this is enough. Then have your friend test your deltoid muscle. It should come as no surprise when it tests weak.

The next phase involves the tester more actively. Tester places three fingers of each hand against your frontal protuberances and holds them there for thirty seconds. All the while, you should continue thinking about your problem.

Your muscle is then retested. It should test strong. If it does not, the holding and stretching procedure should be repeated, perhaps for as long as four minutes. It's just a matter of giving the process enough time.

When at last the muscle does test strong, you will find that your mood has elevated. You will discover that your woes are not as great as you first calculated, and life will seem noticeably brighter.

## BONUS: Instant Relaxation With MRT

The MRT technique we have just detailed can be put to practical use in another manner. You can teach yourself to relax no matter where you are or what the circumstances. You may be surrounded by turmoil, enveloped by chaos; this technique will bring instant calm. And you can do it by yourself.

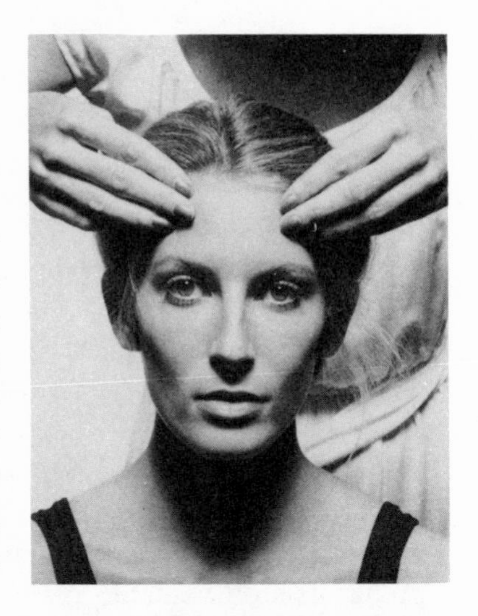

A bit of preliminary work and, of course, some practice are required. It's not difficult, and the reward comes fast and easy.

To begin, pick a number from 1 to 9. Use your favorite number if you have one; if not just choose the first digit that comes into your mind. Also select a color you particularly favor. This combination is your own number/color relaxation pair. Here's how to put them into operation:

Close your eyes and relax as much as you can. Put three fingers of each hand (or the tester's hands) over the frontal protuberances, the bumps on your forehead above your eyebrows. Picture your number against a background of your color. The more vividly you can recreate both of these, the more complete will be your relaxation. Take as much time as you need for this stage, allowing the feeling of relaxation to flow through your body. You will actually be able to feel the tension being drawn from you.

Finally, direct your imagination and your energy to your thymus gland, located in the center of your chest just below the bony notch of your collarbone. Focus your image-making force on this precise spot, but keep your hands in place on the frontal protuberances. Gradually you will feel the stress-relieving capacity of the thymus take over. (If you wonder why this works, read Chapter Ten for a fuller explanation.)

You will emerge from this session, no matter how brief, with a sense of tranquillity and an awareness that the primary impact of the situational stress has slipped away.

You will also discover that the method is habit-forming. Once you have enjoyed the ease and comfort that you can turn on like flicking a switch, you will be hooked. You could hardly choose a better addiction.

CHAPTER

TEN

# Temporal and Thymus Taps

The Temporal Tap is not, in the strictest sense, part of MRT. It does, however, have a shared conceptual basis and the two techniques are frequently used in tandem. Essentially, the Temporal Tap has its most valuable application in the alteration of unconscious behavior. As such, it can contribute significantly to many areas of human concern, perhaps most importantly to the realm of habitual behavior. Are we saying that the Temporal Tap can help you lose weight if you are a compulsive eater or can help you quit smoking if you're a two-pack-a-day smoker? Yes, we're saying that and more.

But first, a bit of background so that the procedure and our claims for it won't seem so far-out.

Many of the inputs to your brain are strained through a logic filter. That's a simple formulation for a much more complex neurological process, but it is an accurate description. The input ranges all the way from auditory and visual communication to unconscious thoughts and impulses, from data you consciously and deliberately seek to the strange, crazy fragments from the dark corners of your unconscious that you try to deny or suppress.

A concept underlying the Temporal Tap procedure maintains that the logic filter is contained within the area surrounding your ears. Anatomically speaking, the area immediately adjacent to your ears contains the greatest concentration of nerves of any portion of your body. A large proportion of the nerve pathways are crammed into the hinge joint of your jaw, the *temporo-mandibular* joint. The focal area for the filtering of sensory input to your brain is the temporo-mandibular joint plus the semicircular area around it, including the bony portion of your skull adjacent to your ears. The theory, again in simplified form, is that the nerve network monitors the informational sensations coming to your brain and allows only certain information to be passed along and acted upon.

The idea of such a filter has a certain basis in observable phenomena. As conscious beings, we regularly employ a process of mental selection. For example, almost any mother can immediately distinguish the cry of her own offspring, even though there may be a room full of screaming children surrounding her own. Virtually every second of our lives, we sort out or strain the total sensory input, winnowing it down to the significant. If we were to remain aware of all the stimuli that are bombarding us, we'd go crazy. We just couldn't cope with that many things coming at us. And so we automatically sort out relevant information, rejecting the irrelevant.

The key to most of it seems to be survival. We are seeking what will help us the most and harm us the least. In one sense, the Temporal Tap is a conscious way of calling attention to some command or idea we want to impose upon the brain.

Physiologically speaking, there are enough holes in this theory to accommodate the entire graduating class of Oxford University. In terms of any framework of scientific analysis, there are wild gaps in the logical progression from cause to assumed effect. Except for one thing: It works. Like the honeybee, who by all rules of aerodynamics is deemed incapable of flight, this procedure does produce the results claimed for it.

Empirically speaking, the evidence in favor of the Temporal Tap is pretty weighty. But again, as with basic MRT, you need not accept any of this on blind faith. Try it yourself. It cannot possibly do any harm; the absolute worst that can happen is that the technique won't work for you. On the other hand, there is a very strong possibility that you will, to your utter amazement, discover a strange new ally in the constant struggle to get the most out of your mind and body.

Now the brain is a pretty savvy organism. It will reject obvious falsehoods or nonsense. It is impossible to impress this sort of information upon the subconscious. For example, suppose you try to tell someone via the Temporal Tap technique that he has three eyes. Even if you should be successful in breaking through the censor, the brain will refuse to accept this statement. Similarly, it is impossible to command yourself, or anyone else, to perform any act that is morally unacceptable. Temporal tapping is not a step away from mustering an army of zombies who will rape, plunder, and pillage.

It is, however, possible to impress upon the brain ideas that are factually and morally acceptable but which the conscious mind of the individual does not believe possible. This is the crux of the Temporal Tap. For example, let's say that you have tried to give up smoking maybe fifteen or twenty times within the past few years. At this stage of the game, you're pretty well convinced that you just can't do it. You may insist that it is beyond your capabilities, but your brain will not accept this assertion for the simple reason that it is *not* a fact. You *can* stop smoking. It is a physical and logical possibility. Your brain firmly believes that you can stop smoking.

It so happens that, via the Temporal Tap, this information can be impressed upon your consciousness. You will, in reality, do what is good for you, although you do not believe it is possible to carry it out. In this, as in most other things in life, the primary limitations that we accept are those we impose upon ourselves. Quite frequently, they have little relationship to reality.

A great deal of investigative work on the Temporal Tap was conducted by Robert E. Ornstein, Ph.D. In his book *The Psychology of Consciousness* Dr. Ornstein says, "Since we construct our ordinary world around the limited input from our sensory systems, we remain largely unaware of much of our immediate environment, either because we lack the receptive organs or because the phenomena change slowly."[7]

This does not have to be so. As we become informed about the subtle forces that surround us and of the significant effects they can have upon our lives, we are discovering that we can boost our own awareness. This means, in part, that we can, to an astounding degree, control not only our bodies but our minds. The probing has just begun.

## The Temporal Tap Procedure

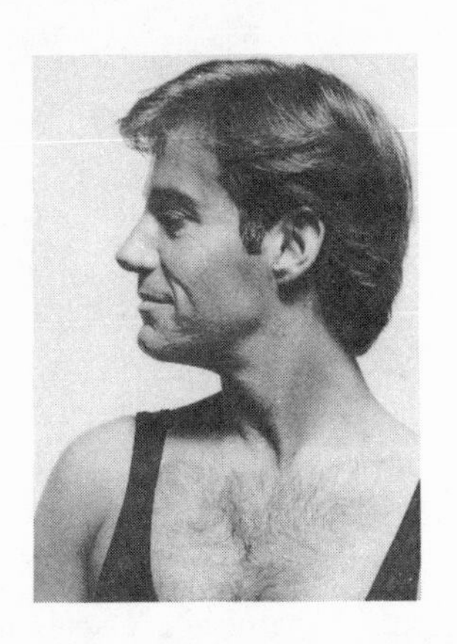

As a technique the Temporal Tap is no big deal. You can do it on yourself or have a friend do it for you. Use the three middle fingers of your hand and contact your head with the finger pads. Tap rapidly in a rhythm of two beats a second. It's a fairly firm beat generated by wrist action.

Where you tap and what path you follow is of signal importance. Begin just forward of the ear. You can locate the exact spot by holding your fingers in the approximate area and wiggling your jaw. As you shift your fingers slightly, you will come upon a hollow area that is just forward of your ear and about a third of the way down from the top of it. The path starts at this spot and follows upward and around the general contours of your ear, about half an inch out from it. If you feel this area, you'll notice there is a ridge of bone in your skull that pretty well duplicates the curve of your ear. The tapping should be done on this ridge of bone.

Follow it all the way around to the spot where your neck comes up and meets your skull. The mastoid bone tapers down to a roundish point here; that is the end point for the tapping pattern. You start just in front of the ear and go over the top of it to the back, where the bone ends.

Regardless of whether you tap yourself or have someone else

do it for you, there is a rigid rule about which hand taps which ear. Suppose you are doing it to yourself. You match hand to ear, tapping your right ear with your right hand, left ear with left

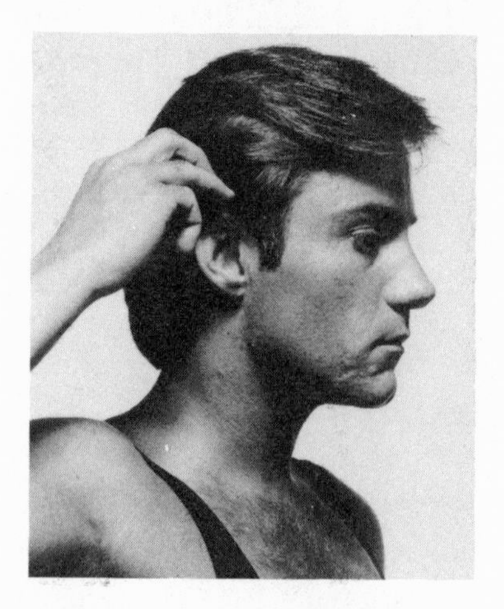

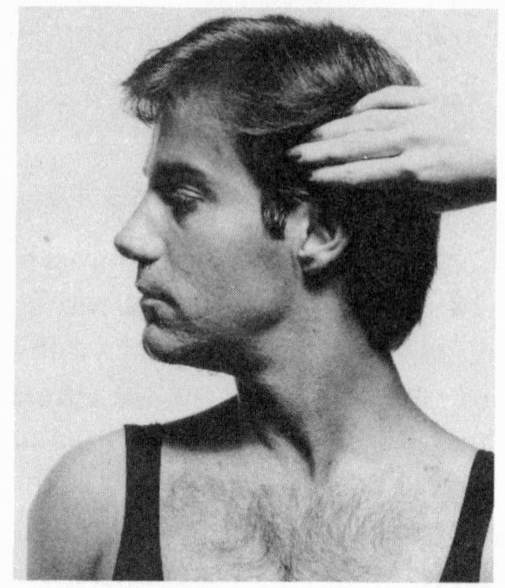

hand. If someone else is tapping, he uses opposite hands: right hand to left ear, left hand to right. This is easy to keep straight if you stand facing each other. The point is that in neither case does the arm have to pass across the face.

Remember, the tapping is a *rapid* series of smart thunks with the pads of the fingers. Keep tapping at the rate of approximately two beats per second as you move your hand in the prescribed pattern around the ear.

What's this all about? Sounds pretty weird and more than a little unlikely. It's not, though. You are probably aware that researchers inquiring into the nature of the human brain have determined that the left and right sides of the brain have different functions and deal with distinctly different areas of thought and action. It happens that the left side of the brain will accept information formulated in a positive manner, the right side will accept information formulated in a negative manner. Remember the filter? Well, if you want the input you have selected to pass through the filtering mechanism, you must slip it in the proper door and in the proper form.

Let's take a moment to define our terms. "Negative" and "positive" are not value judgments here. We are not talking about "good news/bad news" or anything like that. Rather they are grammatical structural factors. "I am alive" and "I am not dead" mean the same thing, but one is a positive statement and the other is a negative one; the first deals with being, the second with not being. Some other positive/negative pairs might be:

"I feel sated."/"I am not hungry."
"I am content without a cigarette."/"I do not want a cigarette."
"I am happy without a drink in my hand."/"I do not want anything to drink."

The point, it should now be clear, is to frame statements in a manner that is acceptable to the side you are tapping at any given moment. The same idea can be communicated to each side, but the terms in which it is stated must be positive for the left side, negative for the right.

Admittedly, this is a bit much to accept on faith alone, and right now is probably a good time for a bit of proof. As we have said before, we believe that you should have a chance to prove our assertions to yourself, and should remain skeptical until you have yourself experienced that proof.

## The Proof

We have devised a test run to demonstrate how the Temporal Tap works. The demonstration is of the two points we have outlined, the first being that the brain will not accept patent nonsense, the second that the left side accepts positive statements, the right side negative statements, and not the other way around.

The first stage employs the Temporal Tap as the means for supplying input to the brain and uses our old friend MRT to indicate whether the brain has accepted the statement. As always, MRT gives a yes or no answer in terms of a strong or weak muscle response.

You will need a friend to do the test with you. Follow the by-now familiar get-ready procedure for MRT.

1. Relax with your test-mate for five or ten minutes.
2. Remove all metal from your persons.
3. Go through the neutralization process.
4. Assume the proper positions: tester standing, testee standing or sitting with legs uncrossed.

The tester should make a determination of the baseline strength of the deltoid muscle, and then, employing the left hand in a temporal tap around the subject's right ear, pronounce a totally absurd statement, clearly contrary to fact, into that ear. For example, "You have two heads." Repeat this three times, tapping all the while. Then retest the subject's arm. It will be weak, which is to say, the muscle is indicating that the brain has said, "No." It simply will not accept that untruth.

Next retract the false statement by repeating three times while you tap, "You have just one head." The arm will test strong, indicating a yes response to the true statement.

The demonstration of the left/right, positive/negative pattern is somewhat more complicated, but it's an interesting routine to try. It's okay, if you prefer to skip this section and go right to a simpler proof. You will need a friend again, this time to compile two separate lists of numbers or words as nearly equal in length and complexity as possible. As these lists are to be committed to memory, they should be longish, but not so long that memorization would be impossible. They should be challenging, but not unrealistically so.

Your friend should begin by temporal tapping two statements on either side of your head. For the first part of the test, utilizing the first of the two lists, the statements should be formulated so as to be *unacceptable* to the brain. That is, he should repeat three times while tapping the left side of your head, "There is no reason why you cannot easily memorize words (or numbers)." To the right side he says, tapping all the while, "You can easily memorize words (or numbers)." The idea here is that the statements may be true, but the formulation is not as required. The left side is told that there is *no* reason and you *cannot;* the right side is given essentially the same message but it is couched in positive terms.

Having administered these messages, your friend should retire with a watch while you attempt to memorize the first list. A record should be made of how long it took you to correctly memorize every item.

The second stage uses the second list, and the input is again administered through the Temporal Tap. This time, however, the rules are followed. Your friend taps the left side and says, "You can memorize words easily," a positive statement; tapping the right side, he asserts, "There is no reason why you cannot memorize words easily." Once again you try to memorize, this time using the second list, and once again your friend keeps track of how long it takes you to get it all down correctly. You may be amazed to find how much more quickly and easily you were able to memorize the second list.

A simpler proof uses MRT and Temporal Tapping in combination. You and your friend should go through the get-ready, as reviewed earlier. Have your deltoid muscle's baseline strength tested. Then you tap and talk while your friend tests the muscle. Tap your left side and say, "My arm is not strong." This is a negative statement and your positive-accepting left ear will have none of it. Consequently, the muscle will test strong. Then tap your right ear and repeat the same statement, "My arm is not strong." In fact, it will test weak. Then reverse it, telling the right ear, "My arm is strong." Nonsense, says your brain, and your arm will translate this to a weak response. Telling your left ear, "My arm is strong," will be greeted with an affirmative—strong—response.

Incidentally, these statements do constitute a valid form of communication, and you can prove this by having your friend make the statements in a foreign language that you do not understand. Even if the proper formulation is presented to the proper side, the response of the muscle will not change. The message did not get through because you could not understand the words in which it was uttered.

Note that whenever MRT is used with Temporal Tapping, the

subject should be neutralized. For Temporal Tapping alone, it's not necessary.

**What's It Good For?**

The possible applications for the Temporal Tap are, it seems to us, endless. As a way to monitor and modify input to the brain, it can be enormously effective in any number of areas of human concern. The most obvious applications are in the area of habitual and compulsive behavior. But some important work has been done in other fields.

For example, dentists are discovering an unusual application in their practice. Some dental patients have a great deal of trouble suppressing their gag reflex. A technique developed by Dr. George Goodheart, one of the outstanding pioneers in the field of kinesiology (the basic science from which MRT developed), can be used to control it.

Dr. Goodheart gives a remarkable demonstration of this technique to doctors in some of his seminars. He touches a blunt instrument to the uvula of one of his students and produces a strong gag reflex. Then he temporal taps on the left side and says to the student, "You'll get along fine without your gagging." On the right side he says, "There is no need for you to gag." On the retest, it's barely possible to get any sort of a gag response at all.

But what can *you* do with this oddball treatment? It is a splendid way to break or change habits you deem undesirable, to free yourself of the tyranny of your compulsions. You make the choices: you can substitute non-smoking for smoking; you can substitute light eating for gorging; you can substitute courage for phobias, trade in unrealistic worries and emerge with tranquillity, swap alcoholism for teetotaling (or any degree of boozing in between). The horizons are truly limitless. Restrictions are few.

One area of restriction does exist, however. You will be completely unsuccessful in ingraining a habit that is morally unacceptable to you. In other words, if you are basically monogamous and that behavior pattern is genuinely comfortable and acceptable to you, you will not be able to Temporal Tap yourself into a Don Juan. It just won't happen.

Temporal Tap can be used, however, to reinforce virtually any habit or action that you *want* to instill. It's all a matter of programming yourself. For example, "I am successful," "I am healthy," "I am youthful," "I am sexy," are only a few of the available possibilities. You can tap those and other positive statements onto the left side of your head; be sure, however, to tap the negative counterpart into the right side. For example, "I am not a failure"; "There is no reason for me not to be healthy"; "There is no reason for me not to be youthful—sexy—whatever."

Because the Temporal Tap is so easy to put into practice, you can use it for a lot of minor inconveniences too. Let's say that you have to memorize some vocabulary lists for a language course that you are taking. Temporal Tap yourself on the right side with a statement such as, "There's no reason why I cannot learn this material easily"; and on the left with, "I can memorize this material easily."

Is your tennis backhand giving you some trouble? Don't have the control you want? Try some Temporal Tapping. "There's no reason why I can't control my backhand swing," goes in the right ear; the left gets, "I can easily develop a strong, accurate backhand."

You get the idea. You should be able to take off from here with a long and happy assortment of useful, strengthening applications of the Temporal Tap.

**Thymus Tap**

In the past ten or so years, medical science has zeroed in on a new enemy in the battle for health and vitality. That enemy is stress, and it has been identified as a continuing factor in a wide range of health problems, from tension and high blood pressure to ulcers, colitis, emotional problems, sleeplessness, weight loss and much more.

It is in the area of relieving stress that a second tapping procedure, the Thymus Tap, has its major application. You may find it worth exploring.

According to Hans Selye, recognized as the world's foremost

authority on the subject of stress, the thymus gland, among its other functions, plays a role in helping your body adapt to and handle stress. Of course, stress greater than your body can bear will show up in the form of ill health. But as a coping mechanism, the thymus turns out to be a first-class ally in the battle against stress. And it is a cinch to use.

The thymus is located about an inch and a half below the bony notch of your collarbone. Here's how to locate it precisely: Starting at the bony notch, slide your finger down the center point of your chest. About an inch and a half below, you'll find a second depression, known as the Angle of Louis. This is the spot where you tap.

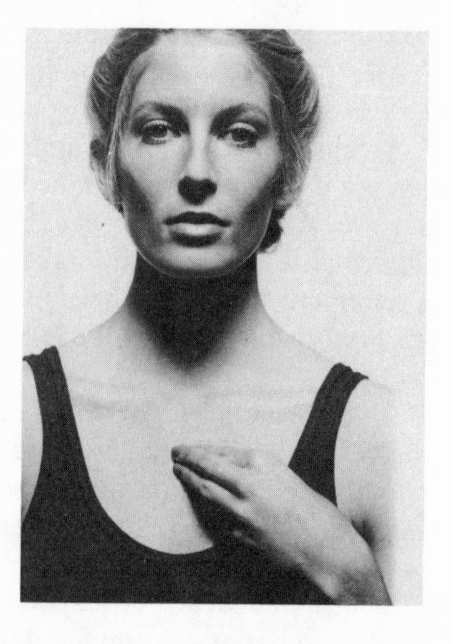

Right hand or left, it doesn't matter. The tapping should be in a brisk pattern of one long and two short taps repeated eight to ten times—da-dit-dit.

No need for statements—this is a silent tap routine and one you do yourself. For a general pepper-upper and tonic, schedule a thymus tap four times a day. Step up the frequency if you find yourself in any sort of a stress-producing situation. If you're nervous, anxious, worried, upset, or troubled for any reason whatsoever, you can sometimes get a gratifying degree of relief by thymus tapping.

Apparently, the brisk da-dit-dit of your drumming fingertips serves to encourage the thymus into greater activity. When this occurs, it helps you cope.

All of which must make it the only no-cost, nontoxic tranquilizer available today.

APPENDIX

I

# Parlor Games

In addition to being a versatile and accurate indicator of your health and well-being, MRT can be a great deal of fun. Once you have become skilled at performing the test procedure and have used it to answer vital questions about your health and those of your family and/or friends, you may find yourself taken with some of the inherent possibilities for showmanship. Employing the basic MRT test procedure and some of its underlying principles, we have devised and collected here a series of stunts that will amaze your friends and liven up any party.

This is by no means to belittle MRT as a valid technique. The games included here all operate on the same principles that serve you so well in your inquiry into your physical health; they work because of the same premise.

A few general hints on how to conduct your performance:

Be sure to practice beforehand. There is nothing so deadly as a bit of stagecraft that doesn't quite come off.

Unlike magic tricks and Ouija boards, there is no mumbo-jumbo, no sleight of hand involved with MRT. There is no need to make it seem more mysterious than it actually is. Explain to your audience what you are doing, keep up a running patter—make it as light and amusing as you are inspired to, but be sure to keep them informed. Tell them what you are doing; neutralize your subject and explain what that involves; announce when you have gotten a weak response, when a strong one; explain how you have altered the stimulus, what you are aiming to achieve. Part of what is truly amazing about MRT is that it works in such a clear and simple way; make sure your audience is aware of that clarity and simplicity.

Do not rush. Follow through the process with the same care and precision you would use in a vitamin investigation. If you try to short-circuit any of the procedures, the whole routine may fall apart.

Some of the test situations we have devised are more reliable than others. We have indicated which may be a little risky. It's a good idea to begin with the sure things; when you have gained the confidence of your audience, you might try some that are less secure. If you find a subject who responds well to any one of these tests, stick with that person; perhaps use him or her on some of the trickier ones. By the same token, if your subject seems less responsive, giving you only moderate reactions, try your next routine on someone else. It's more fun in a party situation to have dramatic demonstrations.

Don't forget to neutralize your subject before you begin. If you do a series on the same person, you need neutralize only once. But each time you begin working with a new subject, remember that he or she must be neutralized.

Begin with a brief speech, explaining that MRT is a muscle-testing system. Then be sure to clarify the difference between a strong muscle and a weak one. And wind up with a simple, quick demonstration that will powerfully indicate the technique. Here's a good one:

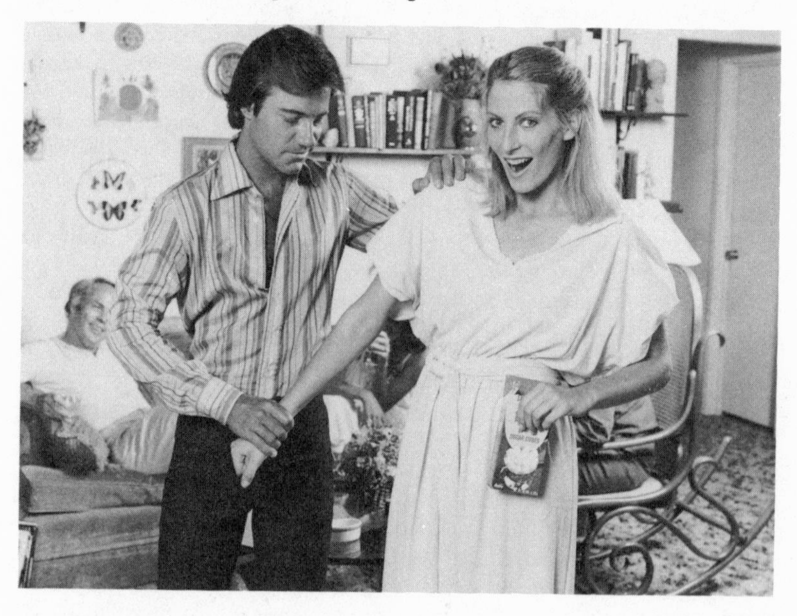

**Sugar and Salt**

From the kitchen, borrow a one-pound box of salt and a box of sugar cubes or a bag of sugar. It doesn't matter what variety: cubes or granulated, brown, white, or raw—it's all sugar. Choose a willing test subject and demonstrate how you test to establish his muscle strength. (Be sure to neutralize him first.) Then have him hold either the box of sugar or the container of salt.

As you know, the results are most dramatic if the subject actually touches the test material. This is fairly easy with the box or bag of sugar. You just open it up so he can get his hand inside. Access to the salt is a little trickier, but perhaps you can have him stick a finger through the spout opening and tip the container enough to contact the salt inside.

Virtually everyone in the world will test weak when confronted with this quantity of either salt or sugar. For indeed, large quantities of salt or sugar are almost universally poisonous. The MRT response to poison is always the same: the muscle gets weak. If obtaining either of these substances is, for any reason, impractical, you can always revert to the large-size aspirin bottle (at least 100 tablets) you first encountered as the learning test in Chapter Two.

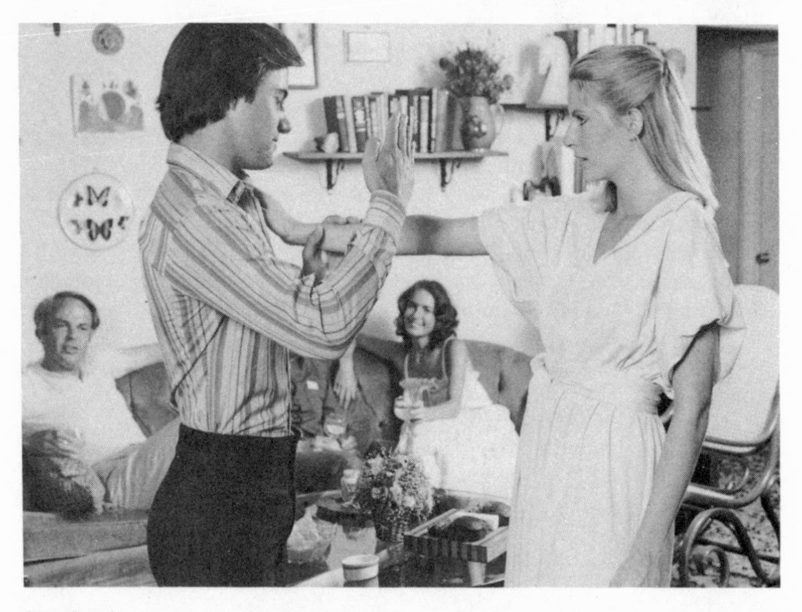

**Cut the Aura**

Here's another demonstration that can be made without a great deal of preparation. The final effect ranges from the curious to the absolutely mind-boggling, depending on your test subject. Since you are now, as you are whenever you practice MRT, dealing with human beings and with human reactions, the process will not be the same all the time.

For this stunt, first test your subject's muscle strength. Then "cut" his or her aura. To do this, extend your fingers rigidly as if your hand were forming a blade. Slice through the air, almost but not quite touching the subject's forearm. Start up above the forearm and continue the action down below it.

The gesture looks as though you were faking a blow against the arm with your outstretched fingers. Repeat this action four or five times in rapid succession.

Retest the subject. The arm will be weak. The only explanation you can offer is the simple, unembellished truth: you have cut the subject's aura. When one's aura is cut, one automatically loses strength. Make certain to reassure your subject. Strength will return in just a moment or two, and you can prove this fact by testing once more.

**Rock the Muscle**

Pick out a hard-driving rock record. It's important that the beat be clearly defined; simple, rhythmic rock seems to work best. Let the subject listen to the rock music for ten or fifteen seconds. Test the muscle. It will be weak. Now play any other type of music, as long as it has an entirely different beat: waltz, fox-trot, jazz, even symphonic. Let your subject listen for ten to fifteen seconds and test again. The muscle will test strong.

Why? The underlying reasons are a bit hazy here, but most experts assume it has to be with the fact that a rock beat is fairly close to a heartbeat, but the tempo is different. The heart, in some undefined manner, tries to adjust its tempo to that of the music to bring the two in line. The mimicking effort is very demanding, and that seems to account for the weakening.

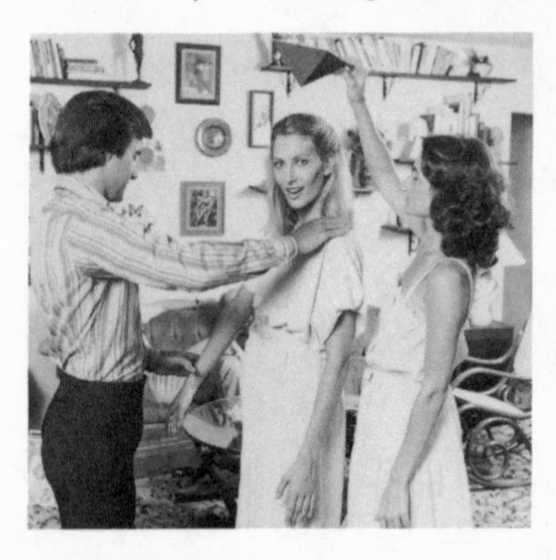

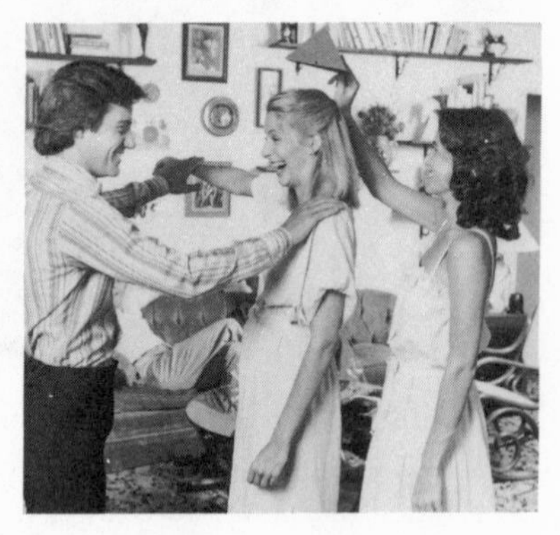

**The Egyptian Effect**

For this one you need a pyramid, one of the small types sold for home use. The open metal framework pyramids are perfectly good; plastic ones are fine; even the cardboard variety is perfectly adequate. You need a third participant, an assistant to hold the pyramid over the subject's head while you test the muscle. Neutralize your subject. Ask your assistant to hold the pyramid point up (as pyramids usually are) or point down. It does not matter which you choose first—when the pyramid is point up, the muscle will test strong; when it is point down, it will test weak. Do the test; then have your assistant reverse the pyramid and test again.

All this might open up another channel for philosophical inquiry. Perhaps, just perhaps, there is something to this whole pyramid business after all.

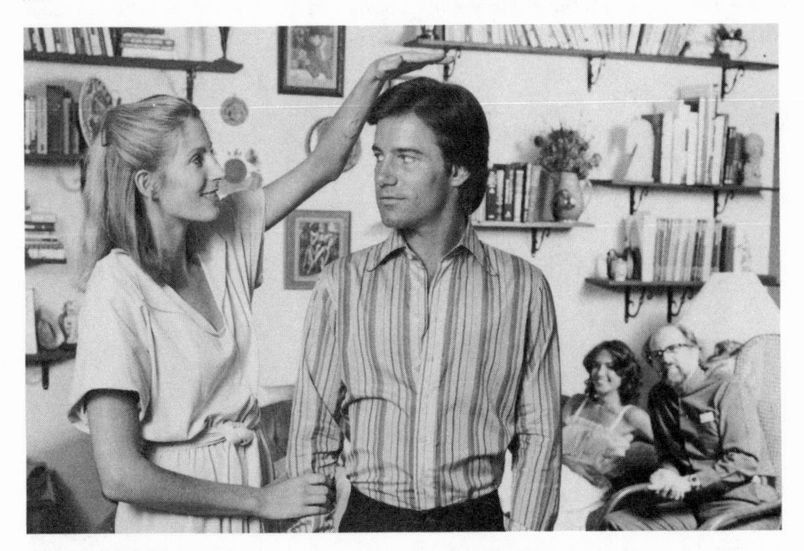

**Sexual Spiral**

Gender differences show up in a lot of different ways. In MRT, responses to certain test conditions will be different—opposite, in fact—depending on whether your subject is male or female. In this parlor game and the two that follow, *Face to Face* and *Hand to Hand,* you can create some audience stunners if you choose a male and a female test subject and demonstrate the differences by testing them in tandem. Just be sure you keep the responses straight and keep up a running commentary so your audience can follow what is happening. And don't forget to neutralize *both* subjects.

Hold your hand just above the subject's head, not quite touching it. Keep your hand palm down during this entire maneuver. If your subject is a female, rotate your hand in a counterclockwise spiral for fifteen seconds; then test her muscle. It will test weak. Reverse the rotation to clockwise and retest. The muscle will be strong. A male subject will give you the opposite response: a clockwise spiral will weaken the muscle; a counterclockwise one will make it strong.

**Face to Face**

If the person you are testing is a man, position a woman about two feet away from him and facing him. His muscle will test strong. Have the woman maintain the same distance, but turn her back to the man. His muscle will immediately weaken.

Try it with a female subject and a male assistant and you will get the opposite result. When the male stands facing the female subject, her muscle will test weak; when he stands with his back to her, it will test strong.

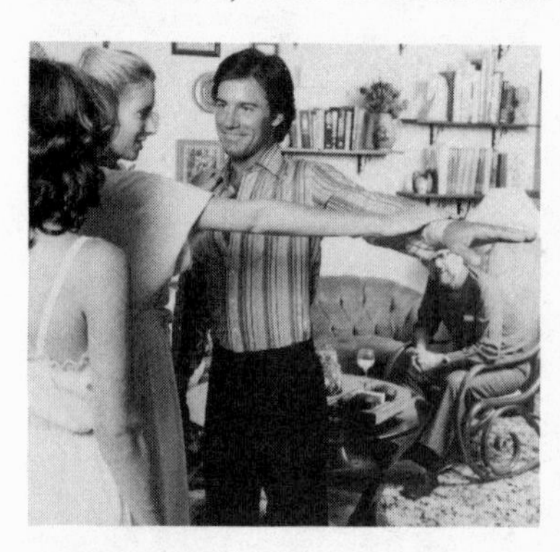

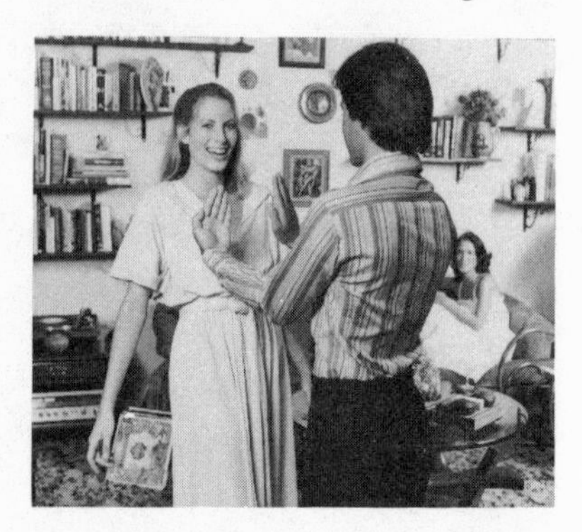

**Hand to Hand**

Stand facing your subject with your hands held out toward him about two or three inches from his chest. The palm of one hand should face the subject, the other palm should face away from him. Hold your hands in this position for about fifteen seconds, during which you call attention to the particular positioning of your hands. Then test the subject and note whether his muscle is strong or weak.

Reverse the position of your hands: the hand that was formerly palm side toward the subject is turned so that the back of it faces him; the other hand is palm side facing him. Maintain this position for about fifteen seconds, then retest. If the subject tested strong before, he will now test weak, and vice versa.

Use a female subject and the hand position that produced a weak response in your male subject will yield a strong response; the position that made his muscle strong will make hers weak.

**True or False**

Have your subject place the thumb and middle finger of one hand firmly against his frontal protuberances (the two bumps in the middle of the fore-

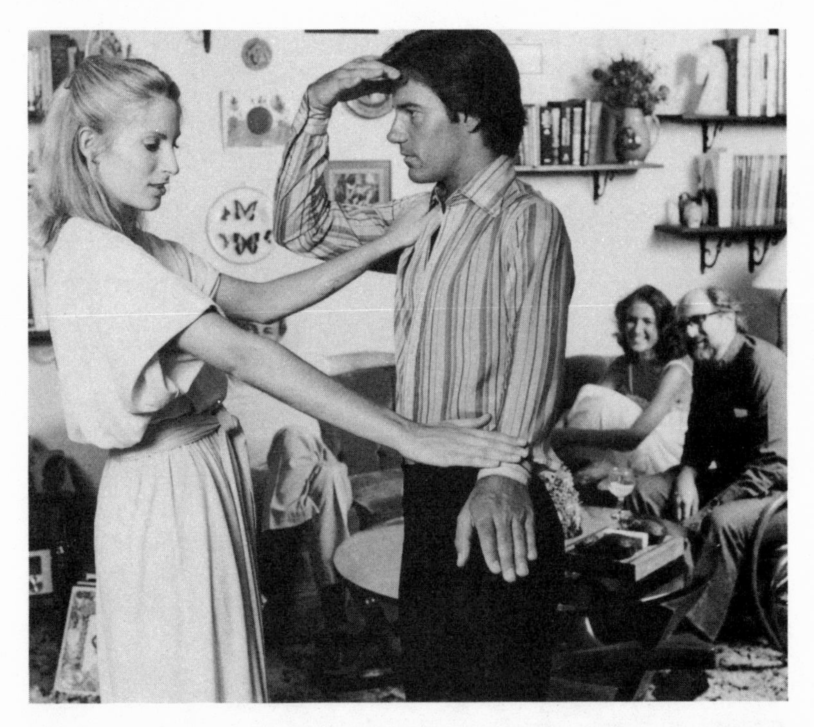

head, up from the eyes and midway between brow and hairline). While he keeps his hand in this position, you make a series of statements and test the muscle of his other arm after each one. You should be prepared with some simple, direct announcements that are flat-out wrong. For example, on a dry day you might say, "It is pouring rain outside this house right now," or to someone in his mid-years, "You are nine years old today." In each of these instances, the muscle will test weak.

Now shift to the truth. Instead of a false statement, announce something that is a simple fact. This could be something like, "Your first name is John," or even, "You are married to Mary." It doesn't matter what you say as long as you keep it simple and truthful. Now the muscle will test strong.

### Telegraph

This stunt is closely related to *Rock the Muscle,* but because you don't need any props, it's easier to demonstrate. Using the tips of your fingers, tap out a rhythm on your subject's sternum (that bony section in the center of the upper chest), what we've been calling the breastbone.

There are only two rhythms you have to learn. If you tap out a dit-dit-da pattern—two short beats and one long beat—five or six times and then test the subject, the muscle will be weak. Reversing the pattern to da-dit-dit—one long beat followed by two short ones—repeated five or six times will make the muscle test strong.

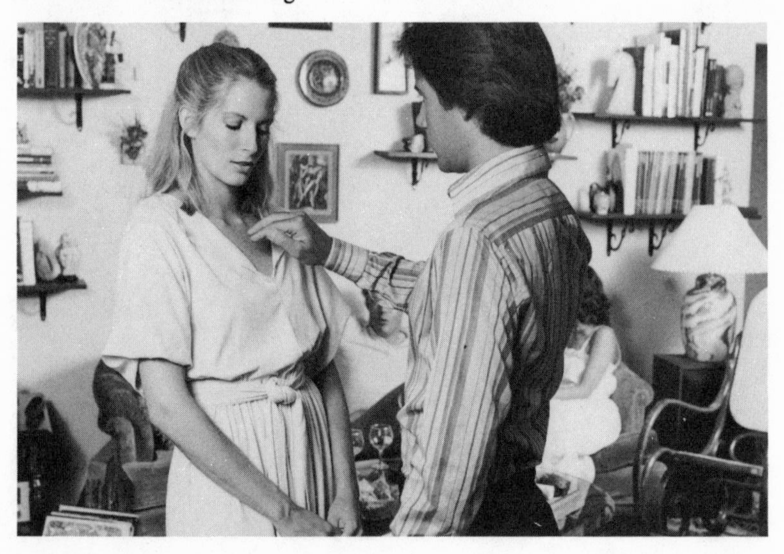

**Friend or Foe**

Ask your subject to place the thumb and middle finger of one hand against his frontal protuberances (the two bumps on his forehead halfway between his eyebrows and hairline). Ask him to think of someone he likes or admires very strongly. Give him ten seconds to concentrate on this individual, then test the muscle of his other arm. The MRT response will be strong.

Then try the reverse: Ask him to think of someone he dislikes intensely. Give him a ten-second concentration period and retest the muscle. This time around it will be weak. Be sure he keeps one hand on his forehead while you test the muscle of the other arm.

You can do a variation on the same routine by suggesting that he concentrate on a person you name. You might choose someone who has been in the news and holds political views you know to be opposite those of your subject; or you can choose a movie star you know your subject particularly admires. The chances are good the subject's muscle will weaken when he thinks about the person with whom he holds differing views and will remain strong when he thinks about the one he admires. In this variant, the test reveals whether your subject likes or dislikes specific people.

**Criss-Cross**

Responses are not always absolute with this particular game, so use it with discretion. To improve your chances of success, work with someone who has responded well to some of the other games we've described thus far. If you've not been working together immediately before trying this one, neutralize your subject first.

The procedure itself is very simple. Seat the subject in a straight chair. Ask him to cross his legs in one direction (either way, it doesn't matter) and test the deltoid muscle. It will be either strong or weak. Then ask him to cross his legs in the other direction. If the muscle was weak the first time, it will be strong now, and vice versa.

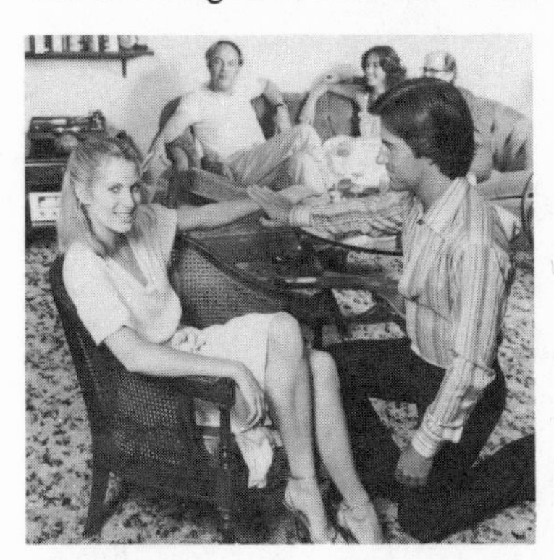

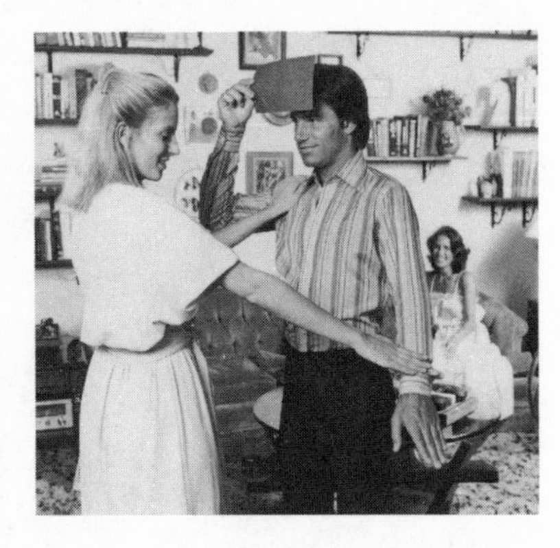

**Color Band**

Get a piece of paper or cardboard about a foot square that is a pure, true, strong orange color. Art stores carry this sort of thing. Look for paper colored on both sides. If all you can find is one-sided colored paper, it should be held with the color facing *away* from the subject. Ask your subject to hold the colored square at the level of his groin. Test the muscle after about ten seconds. It will be strong. Ask the subject to move the colored square to the level of his forehead. Wait ten seconds, then test the muscle; it will be weak.

There is an explanation you can give for this particular phenomenon, but it's debatable whether it would be considered credible in all circles. Those who have delved a bit into the paranormal are aware that, according to one system of belief, there are windows of energy called *chakras* at various points in the body. Each one of these is said to react to a different color.

The color for the chakra for the genital-anal area of the body is orange. When a color is held in position against its proper chakra, the body picks up strength; that's why the muscle tested strong when the orange square was held at the groin level. When a color is held against a chakra that is far removed, such as the head, and has a very different color (in this case it's indigo), the body and, consequently, the muscle lose strength.

**Strong Colors**

Here's another color routine, but with a different twist. Ask your subject what his favorite color is. Hold up anything of this exact color in front of him. It can be colored paper, a scarf, a book, whatever. His MRT will be strong. Now ask him to name a color he particularly dislikes. Again find an object of this color and have him gaze at it for about ten seconds. When you retest, the muscle will be weak.

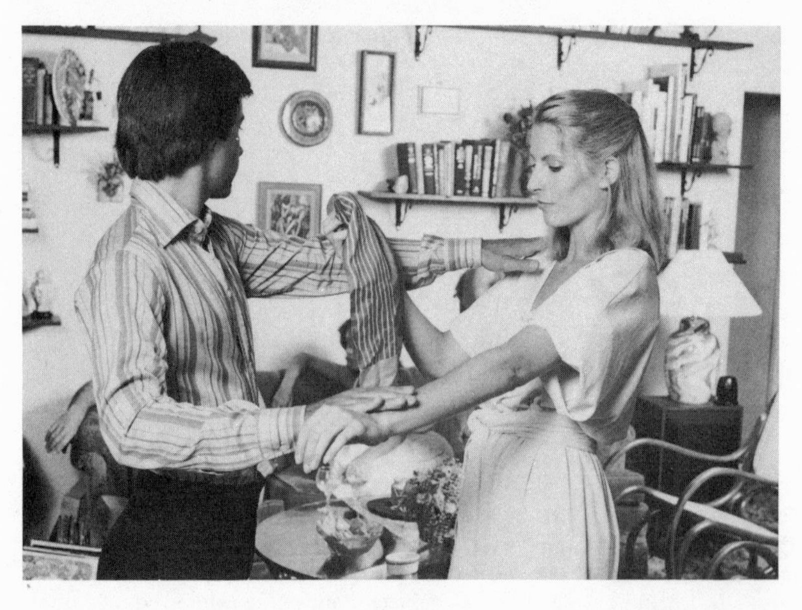

This seems to be a fairly standard reaction. The colors we like are those with which we are harmonious, the ones that enhance or strengthen us. The colors we dislike tend to take away our strength—good reason for disliking them.

**Orange Power**

A word of caution on this one: It works only on men and only with a sheet of paper or cardboard that is a bright, pure, clear orange. Hold this up and have your subject look at it for about ten seconds. In almost every instance, his muscle will be weak. Take away the colored paper and substitute with one of any other color. His MRT response should be strong.

Because the results are not 100 percent guaranteed, this is not a good demonstration to use early on. Here's what's happening and why it's a bit iffy. It is theorized that the weakening of muscle reflects a reaction involving the carotin in the pigmented layer of the eye with that particular shade of orange. Presumably, women do not have the same degree or intensity of pigmentation in their eyes. There hasn't been any real research done in this area, however, so you will be winging it largely on unsubstantiated theory. All we can say is that this particular experiment does seem to work *most* of the time, *as long as the subject is male.*

It's perfectly legitimate to explain that this particular demonstration will not work on everyone and so you may have to try a few people before you can locate a suitable subject. Be warned: this is not a good one to select if you're wagering results against drinks for the house.

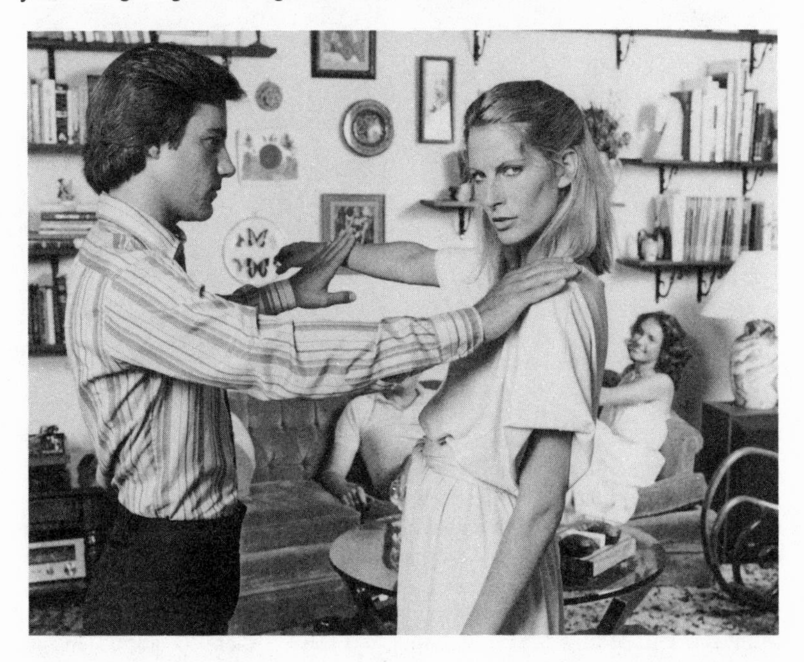

**When You're Smilin'**

Have the subject frown—a deep, full, intense, angry frown that screws up his face. His muscle will test weak. Then ask him to smile—a full, rich, warm smile. The muscle will test strong.

**Mirror-Mirror**

Get a small, one-sided hand mirror. Ask the subject to think of some feature of his face that he likes—eyes, hair, chin, teeth, whatever. Hold up the mirror so that he can see himself in it. With your other hand, test the muscle; it will be strong. Turn the mirror over so that the back faces the subject and retest. The muscle will be weak.

Or try the negative approach: Ask your subject to think of a facial feature he really dislikes. This time around when the mirror faces him, his muscle will be weak; when the back of the mirror is toward him, the muscle will be strong.

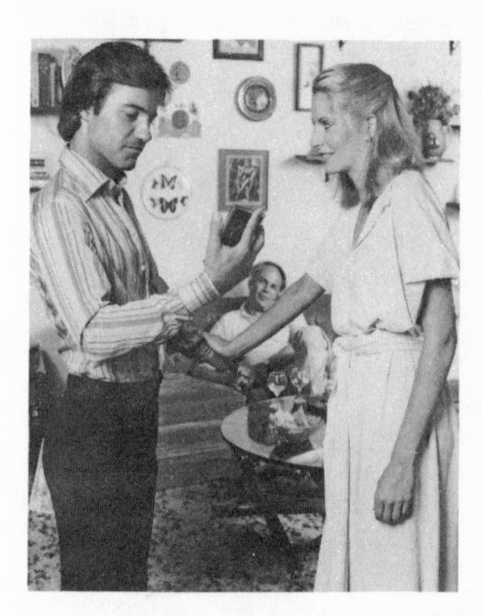

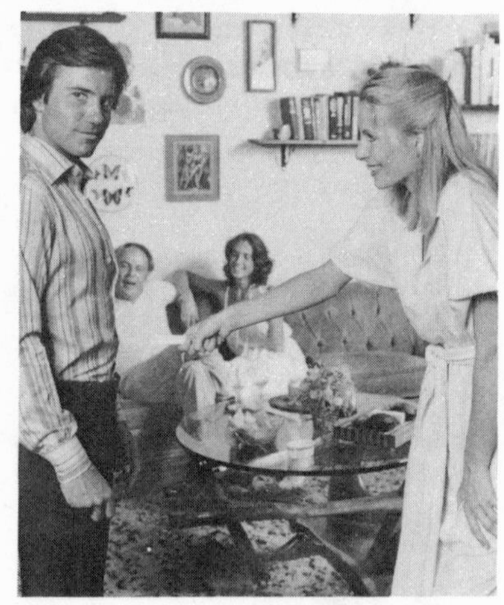

**Magnetic Attraction**

For this game find a subject who has a small, painful area somewhere. It could be a tooth that's aching, a bump, a bruise, a slight headache, or some similar minor complaint. You also need as strong a bar magnet as you can find. (As the name indicates, a bar magnet is straight rather than horseshoe shaped.)

Hold the magnet in your fist with all of your fingers curled around it. Point one end of it at the painful spot and leave it there for about ten seconds. Then test the indicator muscle. It will be either strong or weak. Reverse the magnet so that the other end points toward the trouble spot. Be sure your fingers are wrapped around it and that you point it toward the subject for the same length of time. This time the muscle response will be the opposite of what it was the first time around.

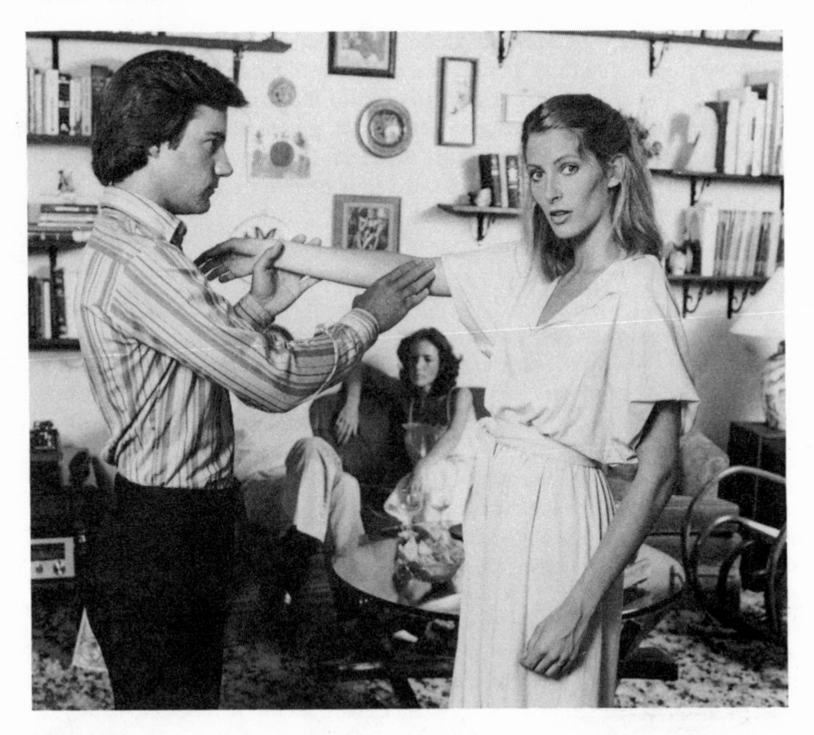

**Run the Meridian**

As we explained back on page 72, the meandering rows of acupuncture points known as meridians can be used as pathways for strengthening or weakening the body as a whole. The test muscle can, as always, be used as an indicator of that effect. The Lung Meridian, which extends from shoulder to thumb along the inside of the arm, is the most accessible channel to use and is particularly convenient because it runs through the muscle we've been using. The strengthening effect takes place when the meridian is followed from the shoulder outward toward the thumb. Stroke lightly with your fingertips three or four times, being certain to lift your fingers from the subject's skin when you reach the end of the thumb and carry them back to the shoulder. Test the muscle: it will be strong. To get a weak response, reverse the direction of the strokes, moving from the thumb up toward the shoulder three or four times. The procedure works most reliably if you contact the skin directly, but you will usually get a good response through one or two layers of clothing.

There is a variation of this technique that verges on the mind-boggling. If the subject is relatively sensitive; that is, if he has responded well to a couple of the other games in this chapter, you might try him on this. Don't touch his body at all. Instead, just trace the direction of the meridian with your eyes. Close your eyes when you reach the end point, reopen them when you begin a new run. Do this four or five times, then test. Then reverse the direction of your eye movements, tracing backward four or five times. Again test. The response should be the opposite.

**North Pole–South Pole**

Get a bar magnet, one marked with the north pole at one end and the south pole at the other. The more powerful the magnet, the better. Hold it in your fist with your fingers curled around it. Position one pole almost touching your subject's ear; with your other hand, test the subject's arm muscle on the other side. Observe whether it is strong or weak.

Reverse the poles of the magnet, again holding it in your fist and positioning it so it almost touches the subject's ear. (Do not change body sides, just change magnet poles.) When you retest, the muscle strength will be the opposite of what it was the first time.

MRT is a valuable tool as regards your health and well-being, but it's also a demonstration of some laws of nature that are not well understood at the present time. As such, it can be used to amaze and amuse your friends. With a bit of showmanship and a dollop of imagination, you will be able to have a lot of fun with MRT. Once you have grasped the underlying premise, you will probably come up with some variations of your own. As far as we can tell, there is no end to the possibilities.

APPENDIX

II

# Vitamins and Minerals

In the pages that follow we have not attempted to list every vitamin and mineral available in every food source or tablet on the face of the earth. The fact is that solid information about vitamins, minerals, and other nutritional elements is remarkably scant in view of the important role they play. We have chosen to list, therefore, only those items for which there is an established or at least a generally recognized value in human nutrition, and we have gathered together from numerous sources what information is known about each. It is our intention that you use this appendix as an adjunct to the MRT tests for vitamins and minerals. The appendix will tell you what the various nutrients are, what they are good for, and where you can obtain them; MRT will tell you if you need them and, if so, how much.

A word about the terminology we have used. Each entry begins with two dosages: *RDA* and *therapeutic*. RDA stands for Recommended Dietary Allowance and it represents the amount of a particular substance the *average* person would need daily to prevent a deficiency state, all other things being equal. In short, RDA is a vague and general measure relating to the borderline between malnutrition and an "adequate" diet. Therapeutic dosage includes larger quantities that various nutritionists and doctors have indicated they have found useful (and not harmful) in improving certain conditions in certain people. We do not intend that you consider either of these two dosages as a prescription for your personal nutrition program. That's where MRT comes in; no need to play Russian roulette with RDAs or anyone else's idea of proper dosage. Rather they are here simply as a record of what is generally considered to be the parameters of possible dosages.

The items listed under the heading *Combining factors* are vitamins, minerals, and other edible substances known to have a beneficial effect on the action of the vitamin or mineral in question. It is recommended that these be taken in combination. Incidentally, aside from Vitamin C, which should be taken at more frequent intervals, vitamins and minerals should be taken at mealtimes or immediately afterward when the stomach is filled with food about to be digested and absorbed into the system.

*Signs of deficiency* and *signs of toxicity* are two sides of the same coin. The symptoms commonly experienced when too little of a particular nutrient is present in the system are listed under *deficiency;* the symptoms evident when too much is present are listed under *toxicity.* In many cases, no toxic effects are known. By and large, this is because excess quantities of the nutrient are excreted in the urine rather than being accumulated in the body. In general, water soluble vitamins and minerals are excretable in this way and there is little danger of overdosing—it's wasteful but not dangerous. The fat-soluble vitamins are passed out of the body more slowly and they tend to be stored in the body as fats, where they can accumulate to toxic levels.

*Possible drug effects* is an important item worth paying close attention to. Listed under this heading are drugs which, when taken in conjunction with the vitamin in question, have the potential to cause problems. (Drug effects are virtually unknown with minerals, so this item does not appear in the mineral section.) If you are taking any of the drugs mentioned, you should consult your doctor before taking the nutritional supplement as well.

## VITAMINS

### Vitamin A

*RDA dosage:* 5,000 IU for adults; 3,000 IU for children
*Therapeutic dosage:* 25,000–50,000 IU
*Beneficial effects:* can reduce night blindness, chronic fatigue; useful in treatment of infections and some skin conditions.
*Signs of deficiency:* night blindness; rough, dry skin; loss of sense of smell
*Signs of toxicity:* nausea, vomiting, diarrhea, hair loss, headaches, flaky and itchy skin
*Combining factors:* Vitamin B complex, Vitamin C, Vitamin D (in a ratio of approximately 1 part to 10 parts Vitamin A), Vitamin E, zinc. When dosage in excess of RDA is taken, calcium and phosphorus should supplement Vitamin A.
*Food sources:* liver, eggs, milk, fish liver oil
*Possible drug effects:* Neomycin, cholesterol-lowering agents, mineral oil
*Remarks:* Vitamin A is fat soluble and is not destroyed by cooking.

## THE B VITAMINS

### Vitamin $B_1$ (thiamine)

*RDA dosage:* 0.5 mg per 1,000 calories
*Therapeutic dosage:* Doctors have been known to prescribe as much as 100 to 200 mg for specific conditions.

*Beneficial effects:* used in treatment of beriberi, herpes zoster; aids digestion, relieves nausea, improves muscle tone.
*Signs of deficiency:* beriberi, fatigue, loss of appetite, irritability, emotional instability (depression), chronic constipation
*Signs of toxicity:* Most nutritionists feel that thiamine has no toxic effects.
*Combining factors:* the rest of the B complex; Vitamins C and E
*Food sources:* brewer's yeast, blackstrap molasses, brown rice, organ meats, eggs, nuts
*Possible drug effects:* Isoniazid, antibiotics, sulfonamides, diuretics
*Remarks:* water soluble.

**Vitamin $B_2$ (riboflavin)**

*RDA dosage:* approximately 1.6 mg for men; 1.2 mg for women
*Therapeutic dosage:* 20–50 mg
*Beneficial effects:* useful for treatment of skin conditions, digestive problems, some eye conditions, mouth sores, burning sensation on tongue, oily skin, premature wrinkles.
*Signs of deficiency:* sores around the mouth (especially in the corners), skin irritations, digestive problems; a persistent feeling of "grittiness" in the eyes, various difficulties associated with the eyes, including extreme sensitivity to light and even some types of cataracts; in severe deficiency situations, retarded growth has been observed.
*Signs of toxicity:* no known toxic effects
*Combining factors:* the rest of the B complex; Vitamin C
*Food sources:* brewer's yeast, blackstrap molasses, organ meats, eggs, nuts
*Possible drug effects:* Isoniazid, antibiotics, sulfonamides, thiazids
*Remarks:* water soluble. Most of the foods eaten in an average diet contain very little $B_2$; this vitamin, therefore, should almost always be supplemented.

**Vitamin $B_6$ (pyridoxine)**

*RDA dosage:* 2 mg for each 100 g of protein consumed
*Therapeutic dosage:* Under certain conditions, as much as several hundred mg have been administered without side effects.
*Beneficial effects:* in treatment of nervous disorders, some blood diseases, male sexual problems, some skin conditions, ulcers, kidney stones, acne, tooth decay; controls nausea and vomiting during pregnancy; some doctors advise it for combating stress.
*Signs of deficiency:* low blood sugar, water retention (especially during pregnancy), numbness and cramps in arms and legs, anemia, nervousness, depression

*Signs of toxicity:* no known toxicity for oral doses
*Combining factors:* the rest of the B complex; Vitamin C, magnesium
*Food sources:* meat (especially organ meat), brewer's yeast, blackstrap molasses, wheat germ, green leafy vegetables, desiccated liver, cantaloupe, pecans, walnuts
*Possible drug effects:* Isoniazid, antibiotics, sulfonamides
*Remarks:* water soluble

**Vitamin $B_{12}$**

*RDA dosage:* 3 mcg for adults; smaller amount for children
*Therapeutic dosage:* Dosages as high as 600–1,200 mcg have been given for nervousness, neuritis, some types of anemia.
*Beneficial effects:* preventing such eye problems as burning sensations, excess watering, and according to some medical nutritionists, even cataracts and some types of diminished sight; helps maintain normal functioning of nervous system; essential for protein metabolism.
*Signs of deficiency:* soreness and weakness in legs and arms; occasionally mental confusion, reduced sensory perception, difficulty in walking, male impotency.
*Signs of toxicity:* no known toxic effects
*Combining factors:* the rest of the B complex; Vitamin C
*Food sources:* organ meats, fish, pork, eggs, cheese and most other milk products, bananas, peanuts, liver
*Possible drug effects:* antibiotics, sulfonamides
*Remarks:* water soluble

**Bioflavonoids**

*RDA dosage:* Not established, although usual dosage is 25 to 150 mg per day.
*Therapeutic dosage:* Some nutritionists have recommended from 50 to 200 mg per day.
*Beneficial effects:* in treatment of varicose veins, hemorrhages of retina and mucous membranes, bleeding gums, arteriosclerosis, eczema
*Signs of deficiency:* susceptibility to bruises; reddish-purple spots on skin caused by capillary fragility
*Signs of toxicity:* no known toxic effects
*Combining factors:* vitamin C, rutin
*Food sources:* green and red pepper, the pulp and white rinds of citrus fruits, raw fruits and vegetables, strawberries, prunes, buckwheat
*Possible drug effects:* none known at this time
*Remarks:* Some researchers feel that it enhances the effect of Vitamin C.

Bioflavonoids are also known as Vitamin P. This material is still under clinical investigation.

**Folic Acid**

*RDA dosage:* 400 mcg for adults

*Therapeutic dosage:* Physicians sometimes prescribe dosages up to 2,000 mcg.

*Beneficial effects:* primarily as a treatment for certain types of anemia; relieves intestinal upset

*Signs of deficiency:* graying hair, frequent stomach or intestinal upsets; poor growth in children

*Signs of toxicity:* no known toxic effects

*Combining factors:* the rest of the B complex; Vitamin C

*Food sources:* dark green leafy vegetables, organ meats, oysters, salmon, root vegetables, milk

*Possible drug effects:* antibiotics, sulfonamides

*Remarks:* water soluble. Because folic acid can tend to mask the symptoms of a Vitamin $B_{12}$ deficiency, it is generally sold separately only in very small dosage tablets. It is considered preferable to take folic acid in conjunction with the other B vitamins in combined tablets, which are formulated with the proper proportion of folic acid to Vitamin $B_{12}$.

**Niacin**

*RDA dosage:* 18 mg for men; smaller amounts for women and children

*Therapeutic dosage:* As part of a magavitamin therapy, niacin is sometimes given in dosages as high as 3,000–4,000 mg per day.

*Beneficial effects:* relieves overall fatigue, muscle weakness, indigestion, skin problems; possibly useful in treatment of insomnia, irritability, and depression

*Signs of deficiency:* canker sores, headache; forgetfulness, depression, irritability, nervousness

*Signs of toxicity:* No toxic effects, but ingestion of large doses can be followed within a few minutes by a brief period (fifteen to thirty minutes) of unpleasant sensation, including intense flushing, tingling, and itching. Although uncomfortable, the effect is not dangerous. If the dosage is increased gradually, minimal discomfort will be encountered, even at the very high therapeutic dosages.

*Combining factors:* the rest of the B complex; Vitamin C

*Food sources:* lean meats, poultry, fish, peanuts, liver, brewer's yeast, brown rice, wheat germ

*Possible drug effects:* antibiotics, sulfonamides

*Remarks:* water soluble. A synthetic version of this vitamin called niacinamide does not produce the same flush as niacin, but it is not as effective as niacin against skin problems and headaches.

**Pantothenic Acid**

*RDA dosage:* none established; various sources suggest between 5 and 50 mg.
*Therapeutic dosage:* Generally from 50–200 mg per day, although amounts up to 1,000 mg have been given without ill effects.
*Beneficial effects:* useful in the treatment of vomiting, stomach problems, repeated infections, hypoglycemia, some circulatory problems, depression, fatigue, arthritis, stress.
*Signs of deficiency:* vomiting, a burning sensation in the feet, muscle cramps, hypoglycemia, allergies, premature aging, asthma, low blood pressure
*Signs of toxicity:* no known toxic effects
*Combining factors:* the rest of the B complex; Vitamin C
*Food sources:* organ meats, brewer's yeast, egg yolks, wheat germ
*Possible drug effects:* antibiotics, especially tetracycline; sulfonamides
*Remarks:* water soluble

Three other members of the B complex—biotin, choline, and inosital—are generally included in combination B vitamin tablets in the proper dosages. They are available in the same food sources as the other members of the B group and share many of the same characteristics.

**Vitamin C (ascorbic acid)**

*RDA dosage:* 45 mg for adults
*Therapeutic dosage:* Dr. Linus Pauling advises 2,500–10,000 mg per day for adults.
*Beneficial effects:* in treatment of colds, skin conditions, anemia (from iron deficiency), stress; promotes wound healing, strengthens blood vessels; sometimes recommended for relief of arthritic or joint pain; possibly of value in lowering cholesterol count.
*Signs of deficiency:* bleeding gums and other mouth problems, chapped and cracked lips, scurvy, excessive bruising, painful joints, anemia, frequent infections, slow healing of wounds
*Signs of toxicity:* Dosages between 5,000 and 15,000 mg per day have been known to cause painful urination, flatulence, loose bowels, and skin rashes.
*Combining factors:* calcium (especially when high dosages of Vitamin C are taken); magnesium

*Food sources:* citrus fruits, rose hips, tomatoes, green peppers
*Possible drug effects:* aspirin and many other pain relievers, tetracycline
*Remarks:* water soluble. This vitamin is readily absorbed and the excess quickly excreted. For this reason it should be taken in a series of doses spread out over the entire day.

**Vitamin D**

*RDA dosage:* 400 IU for adults
*Therapeutic dosage:* 1,500–2,800 IU daily
*Beneficial effects:* useful in treatment of rickets; possibly for some eye conditions; strengthens teeth and gums.
*Signs of deficiency:* soft or weak bones; muscle numbness or tingling
*Signs of toxicity:* frequent urination, nausea, vomiting, muscle weakness, extreme fatigue
*Combining factors:* Vitamin A in a ratio of ten parts Vitamin A to one part Vitamin D; Vitamin C; calcium; phosphorus
*Food sources:* such fish as sardines, herring, and salmon; fish oil, egg yolks, liver, heart, bone meal
*Possible drug effects:* Neomycin, some drugs used to lower cholesterol level, mineral oil, glutethimide
*Remarks:* Fat soluble. Calcium and phosphorus must be taken in conjunction with Vitamin D or it will have virtually no effect.

**Vitamin E**

*RDA dosage:* 15 IU for men; 12 IU for women
*Therapeutic dosage:* Up to 2,000 IU have been used without ill effects for certain conditions.
*Beneficial effects:* strengthens muscles (especially the heart), dilates the blood vessels; this combination helps to prevent heart disease and relieve angina pectoris. Relieves some muscle spasms, aids in healing burns, and is sometimes recommended to dissolve scars. Considered effective for retarding the aging of skin. Can be used as a topical ointment for cuts, itching, and burns. Relieves some symptoms of menopause, bursitis, and arthritis. Some physicians consider it effective against virus infections, and especially flu. Has been used to treat diabetes, phlebitis.
*Signs of deficiency:* gastrointestinal disease, anemia, water retention, heart and kidney problems
*Signs of toxicity:* considered nontoxic, but special precautions are advised for individuals with high blood pressure or chronic rheumatic heart disease.
*Combining factors:* Vitamin A, the B complex, Vitamin C, manganese.

*Food sources:* cold-pressed oils, eggs, wheat germ, organ meats, desiccated liver, leafy vegetables

*Possible drug effects:* Neomycin, some drugs used to lower cholesterol levels, mineral oil

*Remarks:* fat soluble. If both iron and Vitamin E are being included in the same program, the entire dosage of Vitamin E should be taken early in the day, the entire dosage of iron late in the day. Unless they are separated by 8–12 hours, they tend to cancel out each other.

**Vitamin F (linoleic acid)**

*RDA dosage:* none established

*Therapeutic dosage:* In general, 1–2 percent of the total daily caloric intake.

*Beneficial effects:* helpful in treatment of ulcers (especially of the leg) and some skin ailments, such as eczema and psoriasis; regeneration of the skin. Because it plays a role in metabolizing cholesterol, it is regarded by some nutritionists as effective in preventing heart disease.

*Signs of deficiency:* brittle, dull hair; soft or ridged nails; tendency toward allergic conditions, diarrhea, gallstones, acne, eczema, prostate disorders, loss of sense of smell.

*Signs of toxicity:* no known toxic effects, but overdoses can cause a tendency toward overweight.

*Combining factors:* Vitamins A, C, D, E

*Food sources:* vegetable oils, butter, sunflower seeds

*Possible drug effects:* none considered significant

*Remarks:* fat soluble. This fatty acid is commonly available, along with the other so-called essential fatty acids, in lecithin formulations. It should be taken at the same time as Vitamin E for best effect.

**Vitamin K**

*RDA dosage:* none established, but most nutritionists recommend between 300 and 500 mcg.

*Therapeutic dosage:* Dosages in excess of 500 mcg. should be taken only under the advice of a physician.

*Beneficial effects:* Considered helpful in encouraging blood clotting, and so has been used as a protection against hemorrhage and to ease menstrual cramps. Sometimes administered following certain types of surgery.

*Signs of deficiency:* increase in the amount of time it takes blood to clot, internal hemorrhages, miscarriages, nose bleeds

*Signs of toxicity:* The synthetic version of Vitamin K has a tendency to build up in the blood. This can cause a form of anemia. Overdose symptoms are flushing, sweating, and a feeling of constriction in the chest. Natural Vitamin K derived from food sources is stored in the body without any toxic effects.

*Combining factors:* unknown

*Food sources:* green leafy vegetables, egg yolk, blackstrap molasses, safflower oil, soybeans

*Possible drug effects:* Neomycin, as well as some other antibiotics; sulfonamides; some of the preparations designed to lower cholesterol levels; mineral oil

*Remarks:* fat soluble

## MINERALS

### Calcium (Ca)

*RDA dosage:* 800–1,400 mg, depending upon age

*Therapeutic dosage:* up to several times the RDA dosage

*Beneficial effects:* helpful for various problems involving bones and teeth; can alleviate some cardiovascular disorders, arthritis and rheumatism, leg cramps, nervousness, insomnia, headaches

*Signs of deficiency:* muscle cramps, numbness and tingling in arms and legs, porous or fragile bones, brittle nails, joint pains, insomnia, nervous irritation

*Signs of toxicity:* There is no known toxic level from an oral dose; when coupled with a high intake of Vitamin D, however, excess calcium has been known to encourage undesirable calcification of the bones as well as of kidney tissues.

*Combining factors:* Vitamins A, C, D, and F; iron; magnesium, in a ratio of two parts Ca to one part Mg; phosphorus, in a ratio of four to five or two parts of Ca to two parts of P

*Food sources:* milk and milk products, shellfish, bone meal, eggs, spinach, apricots, onions, cabbage

*Remarks:* Always combine calcium intake with Vitamin D for maximum effectiveness. It is important also to boost magnesium intake, especially with the higher dosages of calcium.

### Iodine (I)

*RDA dosage:* .15 mg

*Therapeutic dosage:* Unless derived from food sources, iodine supplements should be taken only under the direction of a physician.

*Beneficial effects:* treatment and prevention of simple goiter; assists in prevention of hardening of the arteries, low blood pressure, listlessness

*Signs of deficiency:* apathy, anemia, goiter, lack of energy
*Signs of toxicity:* impaired thyroid function
*Combining factors:* none established
*Food sources:* seafood, especially shellfish; kelp, swiss chard, turnip greens; iodized table salt
*Remarks:* Regarded as essential in maintaining proper metabolic rate

**Iron (Fe)**

*RDA dosage:* 10 mg for men; 18 for women
*Therapeutic dosage:* Up to five or six times the RDA has been administered in some cases with beneficial effect. Professional guidance is strongly suggested.
*Beneficial effects:* treatment of nutritional anemia (so-called iron-deficiency anemia); especially useful during menstruation; sometimes recommended in the treatment of colitis and ulcers.
*Signs of deficiency:* anemia characterized by lower quantity of hemoglobin in the red blood cells, smaller size cells; pale skin, abnormal fatigue, brittle nails.
*Signs of toxicity:* Long-term ingestion of high doses (over 100 mg per day) has been known to cause toxic effects, including cirrhosis of the liver, diabetes, and pancreatic disorders.
*Combining factors:* Vitamin $B_{12}$, folic acid, Vitamin C; calcium, cobalt, copper, phosphorus
*Food sources:* liver, molasses, kelp
*Remarks:* Excess iron is excreted in the feces and is indicated by a dark colored stool. High intakes of coffee and tea interfere with the body's absorption of iron.

**Magnesium (Mg)**

*RDA dosage:* 350 mg for men; 300 mg for women
*Therapeutic dosage:* Up to five or six times the recommended dosage has been prescribed in some cases, but such high intake should be followed only upon the advice of a professional.
*Beneficial effects:* regarded as effective in reducing cholesterol levels, and in that respect is considered by some as helpful in preventing heart attacks; useful in the treatment of diarrhea, vomiting, nervousness, neuromuscular problems, depression; especially useful to guard against excess calcium deposits in the urinary tract; recommended for preventing kidney stones (especially during pregnancy). In combination with calcium, helps form hard tooth enamel.
*Signs of deficiency:* diabetes, kidney malfunctions, chronic diarrhea or vom-

iting, coronary heart disease, calcium in kidneys, muscle twitch, emotional confusion

*Signs of toxicity:* High dosages (as much as 30,000 mg per day) have been known to produce toxic symptoms, especially in the presence of kidney malfunction.

*Combining factors:* Vitamins $B_6$, C, and D; calcium (in the ratio of one part Mg to two parts Ca), phosphorus

*Food sources:* seafood, meat, nuts, bone meal, soybeans, cereal, grains

*Remarks:* Magnesium is almost always deficient in the average diet. For this reason, most people require a supplement in some form. The calcium/magnesium balance is extremely important. Many nutritionists prefer the supplement available in magnesium oxide over dolomite. Be aware, however, that dolomite contains Mg and Ca in proper proportions; magnesium oxide does not, so if you choose the latter, two parts Ca must be taken with each part Mg. In treating magnesium deficiency, it is advisable to eliminate milk from the diet because it tends to bind with magnesium and carry it out of the body. In general, take magnesium just before or during meals rather than afterward.

**Manganese**

*RDA dosage:* none established; the average American diet provides somewhere between 3 and 10 mg per day.

*Therapeutic dosage:* none established

*Beneficial effects:* helpful in the treatment of diabetes; extremely useful in some neuro-muscular disturbances; encourages production of sex hormones; has a stabilizing effect in skeletal development, strengthening connective tissues.

*Signs of deficiency:* adverse glucose tolerance, poor muscular coordination, ear problems including dizziness and ringing in the ear (tinnitus), anemia.

*Signs of toxicity:* general feeling of weakness, motor problems; there is also a possibility of psychological impairment, apathy.

*Combining factors:* Vitamin $B_1$, Vitamin E, calcium, phosphorus

*Food sources:* whole grains, nuts, beans, egg yolks

*Remarks:* Manganese deficiency is relatively rare. If, however, calcium and phosphorus intake is significantly increased, the amount of manganese should also be increased. People who work in industries that machine or grind manganese are occasionally subject to toxic levels.

**Phosphorus (P)**

*RDA dosage:* 800 mg for adults

*Therapeutic dosage:* When calcium intake is boosted, phosphorous levels should be raised to maintain the ratio of two parts phosphorus to five parts calcium.

*Beneficial effects:* healing of broken bones; cures rickets, eases some arthritic problems, has proven to be quite useful in treating various problems of the mouth, teeth, and gums; increases the effectiveness of calcium.

*Signs of deficiency:* stunted growth, poor quality bones and teeth (lacking strength, porous), arthritis, pyorrhea, loss of appetite, fatigue, emotional disturbances

*Signs of toxicity:* none established

*Combining factors:* Vitamins A, D, and F; calcium (in a calcium/phosphorous ration of 5:2), iron, manganese

*Food sources:* seeds, nuts, grains, seaweed, dried fruit, fish, meat, eggs

*Remarks:* One of the most abundant minerals in the entire body, phosphorus is a major element in the body's chemistry.

**Potassium (K)**

*RDA dosage:* none established; the average person ingests 18,000–25,000 mg per day through a normal diet.

*Therapeutic dosage:* Dosage may be raised gradually and cautiously in the presence of deficiency signs. There is no established dosage.

*Beneficial effects:* controls high blood pressure (if related to high salt intake); effective against some allergies; can reduce symptoms of some types of mild diabetes. Noted as a highly efficient stimulant for nerve impulses, acts to help maintain the proper electrochemical balance of the body.

*Signs of deficiency:* nervous disorders, including such signs of stress as vomiting, insomnia, constipation; low energy level (due to glucose imbalance), general weakness, impairment of neuromuscular coordination, some skin problems

*Signs of toxicity:* no known toxic effects

*Combining factors:* Vitamin $B_6$, sodium

*Food sources:* cocoa, fish, crude molasses, seaweed, dried fruits, most beans

*Remarks:* Highly efficient as a regulator, potassium maintains the proper fluid balance with the body. Supplementary potassium not advised where hypoglycemia and asthma are present.

**Zinc (Zn)**

*RDA dosage:* 15 mg for adults

*Therapeutic dosage:* Can be stepped up to four or five times the RDA without problems.

*Beneficial effects:* Considered useful in reducing cholesterol. Helps speed the healing of tissues, both internally and externally; can increase resistance to infection; considered beneficial in some cases of sexual dysfunction; used in treatment of cirrhosis of the liver, prostatitis; tends to normalize insulin in the blood and so is recommended in some types of diabetes.

*Signs of deficiency:* fatigue, low resistance to infection, mental torpor, slow healing, loss of fertility, some types of skin conditions, diminished sense of taste, white spots on nails

*Signs of toxicity:* Considered largely nontoxic, except in the case of extremely high doses, which may affect the body's ability to utilize the iron contained in food.

*Combining factors:* Vitamin A (increased intake advised when the dose of zinc is raised beyond normal levels); calcium, copper, phosphorus

*Food sources:* organ meats such as liver, kidneys, sweetbreads; fish and shellfish; nuts, wheat germ, brewer's yeast, mushrooms, soybeans

*Remarks:* When insufficient quantities of phosphorus are available to the body, zinc functions at a greatly reduced level.

In addition to the vitamins and minerals listed, there are other nutritional materials that play an important role in the body's proper balancing.

**Ribonucleic Acid (RNA)**

*Dosage:* 30–100 mg; as much as 300 mg is sometimes advised by physicians.

*Beneficial effects:* improves memory; regarded as possibly valuable in recovery from neurological disorders; restores normal thyroid function

*Signs of deficiency:* coldness of hands or feet, coarse hair, low resistance to stress, loss of weight

*Signs of toxicity:* none known

*Combining factors:* proteins; B complex, especially $B_{12}$, folic acid

*Food sources:* fish and shellfish, sardines, onions, brewer's yeast

*Possible drug effects:* phenobarbital

*Remarks:* Experimental studies indicate that RNA may possibly be useful in reversing the degenerative effects of aging.

**Enzymes**

*Dosage:* none established

*Beneficial effects:* aids digestion; increases stress resistance; retards premature aging

*Signs of deficiency:* indigestion, belching

*Signs of toxicity:* none established

*Combining factors:* all vitamins and minerals

*Food sources:* raw fruits and vegetables

*Possible drug effects:* none known

*Remarks:* Aging seems to bring about a loss in enzymes, so some supplement may be necessary. Enzymes are destroyed by heat in cooking, so raw foods are the major food source. Enzymes are also available in tablet form, to be taken with meals.

**Protein**

*Dosage:* tablets: none established (check dosage recommended on brand label); food source: .28 g per pound of body weight.
*Beneficial effects:* primary source of energy; essential building blocks of all cells; vital for growth and development
*Signs of deficiency:* stunted growth, fatigue, anemia, mental retardation, susceptibility to infections, irritability, loss of appetite, water retention, diarrhea or constipation
*Signs of toxicity:* none in normal usage
*Combining factors:* enzymes, hydrochloric acid, calcium
*Food sources:* wheat, fish, poultry, eggs, nuts, milk and milk products
*Possible drug effects:* none
*Remarks: Check with family doctor before supplementing diet with protein tablets.*

***Lecithin***

*Dosage:* 200–1200 mg
*Beneficial effects:* Because of its role in metabolizing cholesterol, combats atherosclerosis, high blood pressure; neutralizes toxity from viral infections; possible assistance in weight-loss programs.
*Signs of deficiency:* tendency toward joint and muscle problems such as bursitis, cramps, and soreness; hypertension; forgetfulness; such digestive problems as intolerance to fat, nausea
*Signs of toxicity:* none established
*Combining factors:* Vitamin $B_6$; magnesium
*Food sources:* soybeans, eggs, liver, wheat, nuts
*Possible drug effects:* none reported
*Remarks:* Some nutritionists feel that large doses taken over a prolonged period of time might deplete calcium levels. For this reason, frequent calcium retesting is advised if lecithin is taken in large quantities.

**Hydrochloric Acid (HCL)**

*Dosage:* 2–3 g
*Beneficial effects:* assimilation of vitamins and minerals, especially iron; formation of bile (for better digestion); improves digestion of protein

*Signs of deficiency:* allergies, some forms of bursitis, anemia, burning sensation in stomach, systemic alkalosis
*Signs of toxicity:* heartburn, nervousness, high blood pressure
*Combining factors:* all vitamins, minerals, enzymes
*Food sources:* apple cider vinegar
*Possible drug effects:* none reported
*Remarks:* Lack of HCL produces the same symptoms as indigestion and the two are sometimes confused. HCL should be taken in pill form rather than a liquid formulation, which can injure teeth.

**Thymus (enzymatic extract of bovine thymus gland)**

*Dosage:* none established, but generally 2–4 tablets per day
*Beneficial effects:* in treatment of skin conditions, infections and inflammations; effective as an anti-stress agent; experiments indicate possible anti-aging effect.
*Signs of deficiency:* none established
*Signs of toxicity:* none established but research indicates possible interferences with antibody production and effectiveness.
*Combining factors:* none known
*Food sources:* upper sweetbreads (also known as neck sweetbreads)
*Possible drug effects:* none known with normal dosage
*Remarks:* may possibly be effective in enhancing thymus-tap effect.

APPENDIX

III

# Allergen Families

Allergy is one of those areas that medical science has made small headway in understanding. Among the things that researchers have observed, however, is that people who are allergic to particular substances seem to have similar allergic reactions to certain others. These groupings, or families, of allergens are worth knowing about if you are embarking on an inquiry into your particular allergy and its causes. The list below of common foods and other edibles will help you by indicating the various related substances to which you can apply the MRT allergy test.*

**Apple Family**

1. apple
   a. cider and juice
   b. vinegar
   c. pectin
2. pear
3. quince
   a. quince seed

**Arrowroot Family**

1. arrowroot

**Arum Family**

1. taro
2. poi
3. dasheen

**Banana Family**

1. banana
2. plantain

**Birch Family**

1. filbert
2. hazelnut

**Brazil Nut Family**

1. Brazil nut

**Buckwheat Family**

1. buckwheat
2. rhubarb
3. garden sorrel

* The following material has been based upon the pioneering nutritional research of Dr. Theron Randolph, and he has kindly given his permission for us to include it in this book.

**Cactus Family**

1. cactus
   a. tequila
   b. prickly pear

**Caper Family**

1. Capers

**Cashew Family**

1. cashew
2. pistachio
3. mango

**Cereal Family**

1. corn
   a. meal
   b. starch
   c. oil
   d. sugar
   e. syrup
   f. dextrose
   g. glucose
   h. cerelose
2. wheat
   a. white & whole wheat flour
   b. graham flour
   c. gluten flour
   d. patent flour
   e. bran
   f. wheat germ
   g. farina
3. barley
   a. malt
   b. beer
4. rye
5. oats
6. rice
7. wild rice
8. sorghum
9. cane
   a. sugar
   b. molasses
10. bamboo shoots
11. millet

**Citrus Family**

1. orange
2. grapefruit
3. lemon
4. lime
5. tangerine
6. kumquat
7. citron
8. citrange
9. angostura

**Composite Family**

1. leaf lettuce
2. head lettuce
3. endive
4. escarole
5. artichoke
6. Jerusalem artichoke
7. dandelion
8. chicory
9. oyster plant, salsify
10. celtuse
11. sunflower seeds
    a. seed oil
12. sesame seeds
    a. seed oil
13. safflower oil
14. cragweed and pyrethrum
    a. vermouth

**Ebony Family**

1. persimmon

**Fungus Family**

1. mushroom
2. yeast
   a. antibiotics
   b. cream of tartar
   c. wine, brandy, champagne, wine vinegar, vermouth, sherry

**Ginger Family**

1. ginger
2. cardamom

**Gooseberry Family**

1. gooseberry
2. currant

**Goose Foot (Beet) Family**

1. beet
   a. sugar
2. spinach
3. chard
4. kochia
5. thistle
6. lamb's quarters

**Gourd Family**

1. pumpkin
2. squash
3. cucumber
4. cantaloupe
5. muskmelon
6. honeydew melon
7. Persian melon
8. water melon
9. Casaba melon

**Grape Family**

1. grape
   a. raisin

**Heath Family**

1. cranberry
2. huckleberry
3. blueberry
4. wintergreen

**Holly Family**

1. mate

**Honeysuckle Family**

1. elderberry

**Iris Family**

1. saffron

**Laurel Family**

1. avocado
2. cinnamon
3. bay leaves
4. sassafrass

**Legume Family**

1. navy bean
2. lima bean
3. kidney bean
4. string bean
5. soybean
   a. oil
   b. flour
   c. lecithin
   d. soy sauce

e. soybean curd, tofu
f. bean sprouts
6. lentil
7. black-eyed peas
8. peanut
a. oil
b. butter
9. jack bean
10. tonca bean
11. licorice
12. gum tragacanth
13. gum acacia
14. pinto bean
15. green pea
16. field pea
17. carob (St. John's bread)

**Lily Family**

1. asparagus
2. onion
3. leek
4. garlic
5. sarsaparilla
6. chives

**Madder Family**

1. coffee

**Mallow Family**

1. maple syrup
   a. sugar

**May Apple Family**

1. May apple

**Mint Family**

1. peppermint
2. mint
3. spearmint
4. horehound
5. thyme
6. marjoram
7. savory
8. basil
9. oregano
10. sage

**Morning Glory Family**

1. sweet potato

**Mulberry Family**

1. mulberry
2. fig
3. hop
   a. beer
4. breadfruit

**Mustard Family**

1. mustard
2. mustard green
3. cabbage
4. cauliflower
5. broccoli
6. brussels sprouts
7. turnips
8. rutabagas
9. kale
10. collard
11. kohlrabi
12. celery cabbage
13. radish
14. watercress
15. colza shoots
16. Chinese cabbage
17. kraut
18. horseradish

**Myrtle Family**

1. allspice
2. cloves
3. guava

**Nutmeg Family**

1. nutmeg
2. mace

**Oak Family**

1. chestnut

**Olive Family**

1. green olives
2. ripe olives
3. olive oil

**Orchid Family**

1. vanilla

**Palm Family**

1. papaw
2. papaya
   a. papain

**Parsley Family**

1. parsley
2. parsnips
3. carrots
4. celery
5. water celery
6. celeriac
7. caraway
8. anise
9. dill
10. coriander
11. fennel
12. celery seed
13. cumin
14. angelica

**Pepper Family**

1. black pepper
2. white pepper

**Pine Family**

1. juniper
2. piñon or pignolia nuts

**Pineapple Family**

1. pineapple

**Plum Family**

1. plum
   a. prune
2. cherry
3. peach
4. apricot
5. nectarine
6. wild cherry
7. almond

**Pomegranate Family**

1. pomegranate

**Poppy Family**

1. poppy seed

**Potato Family**

1. potato
2. tomato

3. eggplant
4. red pepper
   a. cayenne
   b. capsicum
5. green pepper
6. chili
7. ground cherry
8. tobacco
9. belladonna
10. stramonium
11. hyoscyamus

**Purslane Family**

1. purslane
2. New Zealand spinach

**Rose family**

1. raspberry
2. blackberry
3. loganberry
4. youngberry
5. dewberry
6. strawberry
7. boysenberry

**Sapodilla Family**

1. chicle

**Soapberry Family**

1. litchi nut

**Stercula Family**

1. cocoa
   a. chocolate
2. cola bean

**Sponge Family**

1. cassava meal
2. tapioca

**Spurge Family**

1. tapioca

**Tea Family**

1. tea

**Walnut Family**

1. black walnut
2. English walnut
3. hickory nut
4. pecan
5. butternut

**Yam Family**

1. yam
2. Chinese potato
3. sweet potato

**Miscellaneous**

1. honey

*MEAT*

**MAMMALS**

Beef
a. veal
b. milk
c. butter
d. cheese
e. gelatin

Pork
a. ham
b. bacon
Mutton
a. lamb
Horse
Bear
Moose
Rabbit
Squirrel
Venison

## AMPHIBIANS

Frog

## REPTILES

Turtle
Rattlesnake

## BIRDS

Chicken
a. eggs
Turkey
a. eggs
Duck
a. eggs
Guinea Hen
Squab
Pheasant
Partridge
Grouse

## FISH

Sturgeon
a. caviar
Anchovy
Sardine
Herring
Shad
a. shad roe
Salmon
a. red caviar
Trout
Smelt
Whitefish
Chub
Mackerel
Tuna
Swordfish
Eel
Carp
Sucker
Buffalo
Catfish
Bullhead
Pike
Pickerel
Muskellunge
Mullet
Barracuda
Bluefish
Pompano
Butterfish
Harvestfish
Sunfish
Black Bass
Perch
Snapper
Scub
Porgy
Croaker
Mealfish
Drum
Flounder
Sole
Halibut
Rosefish
Codfish
Squid
Haddock

Hake
Pollack
Cusk

### CRUSTACEANS

Crab
Crayfish
Lobster
Shrimp

### MOLLUSKS

Abalone
Mussel
Oyster
Scallop
Clam
Squid

# *Footnotes*

1. Felix Mann, M.B., *Acupuncture, the Ancient Chinese Art of Healing,* William Heinemann Medical Books, London, 1962, p. 2.
2. Harold Burr, M.D. and Leonard Raditz, M.D., "Periodic Changes in Electromagnetic Fields," *Annals of New York Academy of Science,* 1960, p. 462.
3. Louis Moss, M.D., *Acupuncture and You,* Citadel Press, New York, 1966, p. 20.
4. Dr. H. Curtis Wood, Jr., Article in *Prevention* magazine, Rodale Press, Inc., Emmaus, Pa., June 1966, p. 66.
5. Dr. Roger Williams, *Physician's Handbook of Nutritional Science,* Charles C. Thomas & Co., Springfield, Ill., 1975, p. 146.
6. E. Cheriskin, M.D. and M.W. Ringsdorf, Jr., *Psycho-Dietetics,* Bantam Books, New York, 1976, p. 16.
7. Robert E. Ornstein, Ph.D., *The Psychology of Consciousness,* W. H. Freeman & Co., San Francisco, CA, 1972, p. 255.

# Bibliography


Abrahamson, E. and Pezet, A. *Body, Mind and Sugar.* New York: Pyramid, 1971.

Airola, P. *How to Get Well.* Phoenix: Health Plus Publ., 1974.

Aschoff, J. "Circadian Rhythms of Man," *Science* 148:1427, 1965.

Austin, M. *Acupuncture Therapy.* New York: ASI, 1972.

Bagnall, Y. *Nutritional Therapy, A Clinical Presentation.* Wanatchee, Wash.: Nutritional Publications, 1977.

Barnothy, M. *Biological Effects of Magnetic Fields.* New York: Plenum Press 2 vols. 1962, 1964.

Bennett, T. *A New Clinical Basis for Correction of Abnormal Physiology.* Privately published, Burlingame, Calif., 1960.

Benson, H. *The Relaxation Response.* New York: William Morrow, 1975.

Bicknell, F. and Prescott, F. *The Vitamins in Medicine.* New York: Grune and Stratton, 1953.

Bricklin, M. *The Practical Encyclopedia of Natural Healing.* Emmaus, Pa., Rodale Press, 1976.

Brimhall, J. "Mineral Analysis by Hair," *Digest of Chiropractic Economics.* July, 1976.

Broeringmeyer, R. *The Problem Solver—Nutritionally Speaking.* Murray, Ky.: Privately published, 1977.

Bunning, E. *The Physiological Clock.* New York: Springer-Verlag, 1970.

Cheraskin, E. and Ringsdorf, W. *New Hope for Incurable Diseases,* New York: Exposition Press, 1971.

——— ——— and Clark, J. *Diet and Disease.* Emmaus, Pa: Rodale Press, 1968.

——— ——— with Brecher, A. *Psycho Dietetics.* New York: Stein and Day, 1974.

Chipperfield, B. and Chipperfield, J. "Magnesium and the Heart" (Editorial) *American Heart Journal* 93:679, 1972.

Clark, L. *Stay Young Longer.* New York: Pyramid, 1961.

Davis, A. *Let's Eat Right to Keep Fit.* New York: Harcourt, Brace. 1954.
——— *Let's Get Well.* New York: Signet, 1972.
——— and Rowls, W. *The Magnetic Effect.* Hicksville, New York: Exposition Press, 1975.
Dennison, D. and McWilliams, P. *The TM Book.* New York: Warner, 1975.
de la Warr, G. and Baker, D. *Biomagnetism.* Oxford, Delawarr Laboratories, 1967.
Dilling, K. "Applied Trophology." *Nutrition and Public Interest.* Vol. 9. Standard Process Laboratory, Milwaukee, Wisc.: 1965.
Ellis, J. *The Doctor Who Looked at Hands.* New York: Vantage Press, 1966.
Feldenkreis, M. *Body and Mature Behavior.* New York: University Press, 1957.
Frank, B. *Nucleic Acid Therapy in Aging and Degenerative Diseases.* New York: Psychological Library, 1969.
Fredericks, C. and Goodman, H. *Low Blood Sugar and You.* New York: Grosset and Dunlap, 1969.
——— *Eating Right for You.* New York: Grosset and Dunlap, 1972.
Friedman M. and Rosenman, R. *Type A Behavior and Your Heart.* Greenwich, Conn., Fawcet-Crest, 1974.
Goodhart, R. and Shils, M. *Modern Nutrition in Health and Disease.* Philadelphia: Lea and Febiger, 1973.
Goodheart, Jr. G. "Applied Kinesiology." Research Manuals: 1965, 1974, 1975, 1976, 1977. Privately published, Detroit.
——— "Collected Published Articles and Reprints." Detroit: 1969.
Gray, H. *Anatomy of the Human Body.* 27th. Ed., Philadelphia: 1961.
Haimes, L. and Tyson, R. *How to Triple Your Energy.* New York: Playboy Press, 1977.
Harper, H. *Review of Physiological Chemistry.* Lange Medical Publ. Los Altos, Calif., 1973.
Hodezby, H. "The Fountain of Youth." *Natural Food and Farming Magazine,* 1966.
Hrachovec, J. *Keeping Young and Living Longer.* Los Angeles: Sherbourne, 1972.
Hunt, R. *The Seven Keys to Colored Healing.* London: C. W. Daniel, 1971.
Inglis, B. *Fringe Medicine.* London: Farber, 1964.
Inyushin, V. *Questions of Theoretical and Applied Biology.* Alma-Ata. Science Publishing, Kazak, USSR, 1967.
Irving, J. *Calcium and Phosphorus Metabolism.* New York: Academic Press, 1973, p. 187.
Johnson, A. *Biochemical Nutrition for Spine, Nerves and Body.* A. C. Johnson. Palm Springs, 1975.
Karagulla, S. *Breakthrough to Creativity.* Los Angeles: De Vross, 1967.

Karlins, M., and Andrews, L. *Biofeedback: Turning on the Power of Your Mind.* New York: Lippincott, 1972.

Kendall, H., Kendall, F. and Wadsworth, G. *Muscles, Testing and Functions.* Baltimore: Williams and Wilkins, 1971.

Kilner, W. *The Human Aura.* New York: New York University Books: 1965.

Kugler, J. *Slowing Down the Aging Process.* New York: Pyramid, 1973.

Leonard, J., Hofer, J. and Pritkin, N. *Live Longer Now.* New York: Dunlap, 1974.

Lilliston, L. *Megavitamins.* Greenwich, Conn.: Fawcett, 1975.

Lowen, A. *The Language of the Body.* New York: Collier, 1958.

Maharishi Mahesh Yogi *Transcendental Meditation: Serenity without Drugs.* New York: Signet, 1968.

Manaka, Y., and Urquhart, I. *The Layman's Guide to Acupuncture.* New York: Weatherhill, 1972.

Mann, F. *Acupuncture—The Ancient Chinese Art of Healing.* London: William Heinemann Medical Books, 1962.

Martin, C. *How to Live to Be 100, Actively, Healthily, Vigorously.* New York: Simon and Schuster, 1967.

Martin, W. *Basic Nutrition Essential for Improvement of Public Health.* New York: Stein and Day, 1972.

Mertz, W. "Trace Element Nutrition in Health and Disease: Contribution and Problems of Analysis." *Journal of Clinical Chemistry.* V. 21. pp. 468–475, 1975.

Morter, Jr., M. "Bio-Energetic Synchronization Technique." *Digest of Chiropractic Economics,* 1976.

Moss, L. *Acupuncture and You.* New York: Citadel, 1966.

Nittler, A. *A New Breed of Doctor.* New York: Pyramid, 1973.

Ostrader, S., and Schroeder, L. *Psychic Discoveries Behind the Iron Curtain.* Englewood Cliffs, N.J.: Prentice-Hall, 1970.

Otani, S. *A Possible Relationship Between Skin Resistance and ESP Response Pattern.* New York: Citadel, 1968.

Palm, D. *Diet Away Your Stress, Tension and Anxiety.* New York: Doubleday, 1976.

Passwater, R. *Super Nutrition.* New York: Simon and Schuster, 1975.

Pauling, L. *Vitamin C and the Common Cold.* San Francisco: Freeman, 1970.

Pelletier, K. *Mind as a Healer, Mind as a Slayer.* New York: Delta, 1977.

Penfield, W., and Rasmussen, T. *The Cerebral Cortex of Man.* MacMillan, 1952.

Pressman, A. *Electromagnetic Fields and Life.* New York: Plenum, 1970.

Repetzsky, L. *Biotelegraph.* Leningrad: Banner, 1967.

Rosenberg, H., and Feldzamen, A. *The Book of Vitamin Therapy.* New York: Putnam, 1974.

Ryzl, M. "Review of Biological Radio." *Journal of Parapsychology*, Vol. 26, No. 3, 1962.

Shute, W., and Taub, H. *Vitamin E for Ailing Healthy Hearts.* New York: Pyramid, 1972.

Solomon, N. *The Truth about Weight Control.* New York: Dell, 1971.

Steiner, L. *Make the Most of Yourself.* Englewood Cliffs, N.J.,: Prentice-Hall, 1954.

Stoffels, H. *Test and Response Research Manual.* Privately published. Porterville, Calif., 1975.

Stoner, F. *The Eclectic Approach to Chiropractic.* Las Vegas: F.I.S., 1975.

U.S. Department of Agriculture Research Service. "Food Consumption of Households in the United States." U.S. Government Printing Office. Reports: 1–5, 1968.

Walter, D. *Applied Kinesiology.* Pueblo, Colorado, Systems DC. 1976.

Watson, G. *Nutrition and Your Mind.* New York: Harper and Row, 1972.

Williams, R. *Nutrition Against Disease.* New York: Pitman, 1971.

# Index